HIV/AIDS

HIV/AIDS

Kathy S. Stolley and John E. Glass

Health and Medical Issues Today

GREENWOOD PRESS
An Imprint of ABC-CLIO, LLC

A B C 🞂 C L I O

Santa Barbara, California • Denver, Colorado • Oxford, England

Library of Congress Cataloging-in-Publication Data

Stolley, Kathy S.
  HIV/AIDS / Kathy S. Stolley and John E. Glass.
      p. ; cm. — (Health and medical issues today)
  Includes bibliographical references and index.
  ISBN 978-0-313-34421-3 (hard copy: alk. paper)—ISBN 978-0-313-34422-0 (ebook)
  1. AIDS (Disease)—Social aspects. I. Glass, John E. II. Title. III. Series: Health and medical issues today.
  [DNLM: 1. HIV Infections. 2. Acquired Immunodeficiency Syndrome. 3. Social Perception. 4. Socioeconomic Factors.   WC 503.7 S8756h 2009]
  RA643.8.S766 2009
  362.196'9792—dc22   2009026066

13 12 11 10 9   1 2 3 4 5

This book is also available on the World Wide Web as an eBook.
Visit www.abc-clio.com for details.

ABC-CLIO, LLC
130 Cremona Drive, P.O. Box 1911
Santa Barbara, California 93116-1911

This book is printed on acid-free paper

Manufactured in the United States of America

From Kathy:

To Billy, as always, and to my professors (most especially Karen, Phyllis, Jay, and Steve) and to Tim and his staff at TACT for your model, your mentorship, and most of all for making a difference. Thank you.

From John:

I dedicate this to the professor whose name I have forgotten, whom in my freshman year of college covered my first written assignment in red ink and then later sat down with me to demonstrate how to properly write a scholarly paper. As painful as it was to endure this humiliation, the lessons learned from his dedication have proven to be invaluable.

CONTENTS

Every day, the public is bombarded with information on developments in medicine and health care. Whether it is on the latest techniques in treatments or research, or on concerns over public health threats, this information directly impacts the lives of people more than almost any other issue. Although there are many sources for understanding these topics—from Web sites and blogs to newspapers and magazines—students and ordinary citizens often need one resource that makes sense of the complex health and medical issues affecting their daily lives.

The *Health and Medical Issues Today* series provides just such a one-stop resource for obtaining a solid overview of the most controversial areas of health care today. Each volume addresses one topic and provides a balanced summary of what is known. These volumes provide an excellent first step for students and lay people interested in understanding how health care works in our society today.

Each volume is broken into several sections to provide readers and researchers with easy access to the information they need:

- Section I provides overview chapters on background information—including chapters on such areas as the historical, scientific, medical, social, and legal issues involved—that a citizen needs to intelligently understand the topic.
- Section II provides capsule examinations of the most heated contemporary issues and debates, and analyzes in a balanced manner the viewpoints held by various advocates in the debates.

- Section III provides a selection of reference material, such as annotated primary source documents, a timeline of important events, and
  a directory of organizations that serve as the best next step in learning
  about the topic at hand.

The *Health and Medical Issues Today* series strives to provide readers
with all the information needed to begin making sense of some of the most
important debates going on in the world today. The series includes
volumes on such topics as stem-cell research, obesity, gene therapy,
alternative medicine, organ transplantation, mental health, and more.

INTRODUCTION

Thirty years ago, the average person knew nothing of HIV/AIDS; she or he had not heard of it and as such, had no reason to fear it. Today, however, the vast majority of people around the globe have heard of it and most, if not all fear even the mention of it. What happened? To put it simply, a global pandemic happened. A potent virus spread throughout the human population initially due to ignorance of its existence and methods of transmission and later due to continued ignorance and human behavior. Today, there are millions of people *infected* by HIV/AIDS, and many more each day have their lives *affected* by it.

So, what do we now know about HIV/AIDS? Translating what medical researchers have told us about it into everyday language, we know that there is no vaccine that prevents HIV. We know that once infected with HIV, medications allow a person to forestall death for a certain amount of time (much longer today than in the past). We know that once diagnosed with AIDS, the infected person's condition deteriorates far more rapidly. Most significantly, we know that currently there is no cure. In other words, HIV infection creates much suffering.

We know also that virtually all persons are or have been affected by HIV/AIDS; in other words, even those not *infected* by HIV and who do not personally know anyone with the virus are still *affected* in many ways. HIV has cut across many of the social lines that typically separate people from one another; most tragically, perhaps, we know that no one is immune from infection, regardless of age, as even newborns can be HIV+.

Fan, Conner and Villareal (2007: 169) stated these last points best:

All of us live with AIDS. Some of us have HIV, others have full-blown AIDS, and still others are HIV negative. Whatever our HIV status, however, all of us, as members of our society and the interconnected world, are living with the realities of HIV and AIDS, either directly or indirectly.

In this book, we explore many facets of HIV/AIDS as an attempt to better understand how we are all affected by this pandemic. Our understanding of HIV/AIDS and its consequences continues to grow. One hopes that one day the pandemic will come to an end and no one will have reason to ever mutter again, "All of us live with AIDS."

REFERENCE

Fan, Hung Y., Ross F. Conner, and Luis P. Villareal. 2007. *AIDS: Science and Society,* 5th ed. Boston: Jones and Bartlett.

PART I

Overview

CHAPTER 1

Overview of HIV and AIDS

In this chapter, we will look at

- Definitions of HIV and AIDS
- Definitions of epidemics and pandemics, specifically as applied to HIV/AIDS
- Theories about the origin of HIV
- The mechanisms of how HIV and AIDS "work" and how HIV is transmitted

For many people, HIV and AIDS are the same thing; they are interchangeable terms for seemingly the same condition. Although the two acronyms are oftentimes used in the same sentence, they are in actuality two different medical issues. Before we can begin talking about either one effectively, we need to first distinguish between the two.

WHAT ARE HIV AND AIDS?

Although we often hear the terms "HIV" and "AIDS" used interchangeably, HIV and AIDS are not the same thing. The abbreviation HIV stands for Human Immunodeficiency Virus. HIV is the virus that causes Acquired Immune Deficiency Syndrome, otherwise known as AIDS. AIDS develops in the late stages of HIV infection.

A person who has been infected with HIV is referred to as being HIV positive (HIV+). An HIV+ person may be asymptomatic, meaning that he may not have any symptoms of being infected. Although there are many negative stereotypes of HIV-infected people, it is impossible to look at someone and tell if he is HIV+. Many people who are infected with HIV may look and feel healthy. Just because a person has been infected with

DOES EVERYONE WITH HIV DEVELOP AIDS?

Some individuals who are infected with HIV, perhaps 1 in every 3,000, do not progress to AIDS, even without taking antiretroviral medications. Their immune system seems to be able to control the virus on its own for decades, although some do eventually decline. This is unusual because most people (an estimated 85% or more) who contract HIV and do not undertake a treatment regimen will progress to AIDS within an estimated 8 to 12 years or so. Researchers identify people in this category by various terms: long-term nonprogressors, elite controllers, elite suppressors, and HIV controllers. Conversely, people whose immune systems are unable to control the virus are known as progressors, or noncontrollers. The term "elite controllers" often refers to the very healthiest of this subset of the HIV+ population. These are people who have a viral load of no more than 50 copies of HIV per milliliter of blood for a year or more.

Researchers have been studying elite controllers since the 1980s to learn why they do not progress to AIDS. Most of these researchers agree that this is not because the strains of HIV that elite controllers have contracted are any different or less aggressive than viral strains contracted by others. Rather, the elite controllers' immune systems somehow function differently than most people's immune systems and control the replication of HIV within their bodies.

Scientists are continuing to devise new studies to learn more about why elite controllers immune systems work so differently. By studying elite controller's immune systems, researchers hope to be able to design an effective vaccine against the virus, find an effective way to stop HIV from progressing, or even find a cure.

REFERENCES

"Insights from People Who Keep HIV in Check Naturally." No date. National Institute of Allergy and Infectious Disease. National Institutes of Health Web Site. Accessed online November 2008. http://www3.niaid.nih.gov/topics/HIVAIDS/Understanding/insightsEliteControllers.htm.

McCord, Alan. 2008. "Elite Controllers May Show Way to a Cure." August 11. The Body Web site. Accessed online November 2008. http://www.thebody.com/content/confs/aids2008/art48375.htm

HIV does not mean that he has or will be certain to develop AIDS. However, left untreated, most people with HIV infection eventually do develop AIDS. Without treatment, the time frame between a person becoming infected with HIV and subsequently developing AIDS is generally eight to ten years. However, there are cases of HIV+ people remaining asymptomatic for over two decades.

As noted, AIDS is an acronym for **acquired immune deficiency syndrome.** This is a **condition** that develops from HIV infection. The full name is an accurate description of what occurs to a body infected with HIV; namely, it results in a *deficient* immune system. AIDS is diagnosed by criteria established by the CDC. The first diagnostic definition issued in 1982 focused only on symptoms associated with diseases associated with immune system failure (CDC, 1982). However, this definition evolved as scientists learned more about AIDS. A more refined definition issued in 1993 is in place at this writing (CDC, 1992).

In the United States, a diagnosis of AIDS is made when an HIV+ person's CD4 cell count (cells that fight infection) falls below 200 cells/mm^3 and the person has one of a list of conditions identified by the CDC as opportunistic infections. As most people know, our immune system is the body's collective attempt to fight off whatever may be compromising healthy bodily functioning (bacteria, viruses, etc.). It is activated when we become ill or have the potential to become ill. For healthy people, it permits timely recovery and healing from illness. When compromised, it results in a reduced ability to fight off infection and increases the likelihood of becoming ill with other diseases. These infections are called "opportunistic" because they take the opportunity to attack when immune systems are immunosuppressed, meaning the immune system is functioning too poorly to fight off the infection. Although we commonly hear and use the terminology of someone "dying of AIDS," people actually do not die of AIDS. What they do die of are these opportunistic infections that overwhelm their bodies.

It varies as to the amount of time it takes for someone infected with HIV to be diagnosed with AIDS. Prior to 1996, most health professionals estimated that 50% of persons infected with HIV would receive a diagnosis of AIDS within 10 years. Variation from time of infection to AIDS diagnosis was due to factors such as the health of the individual, risky behaviors the individual engaged in, access to medical care, quality of medical care received, living conditions, and so forth. From 1996 onward, however, there have been very effective antiretroviral drugs and other therapies that have lengthened the time between infection and AIDS diagnosis. In addition, there have been new medical technologies developed

Opportunistic Infections identified by the U.S. Centers for Disease Control and Prevention in making a diagnosis of AIDS*

- Candidiasis of bronchi, trachea, or lungs
- Candidiasis, esophageal
- Cervical cancer, invasive
- Coccidioidomycosis, disseminated or extrapulmonary
- Cryptococcosis, extrapulmonary
- Cryptosporidiosis, chronic intestinal (greater than one month's duration)
- Cytomegalovirus disease (other than liver, spleen, or nodes)
- Cytomegalovirus retinitis (with loss of vision)
- Encephalopathy, HIV-related
- Herpes simplex: chronic ulcer(s) (greater than one month's duration); or bronchitis, pneumonitis, or esophagitis
- Histoplasmosis, disseminated or extrapulmonary
- Isosporiasis, chronic intestinal (greater than one month's duration)
- Kaposi's sarcoma
- Lymphoma, Burkitt's (or equivalent term)
- Lymphoma, immunoblastic (or equivalent term)
- Lymphoma, primary, of brain
- Mycobacterium avium complex or *M. kansasii,* disseminated or extrapulmonary
- Mycobacterium tuberculosis, any site (pulmonary or extra-pulmonary)
- Mycobacterium, other species or unidentified species, disseminated or extrapulmonary
- Pneumocystis carinii pneumonia
- Pneumonia, recurrent
- Progressive multifocal leukoencephalopathy
- Salmonella septicemia, recurrent
- Toxoplasmosis of brain
- Wasting syndrome due to HIV

REFERENCE

Centers for Disease Control and Prevention (CDC). 1992. "1993 Revised Classification System for HIV Infection and Expanded Surveillance Case Definition for AIDS Among Adolescents and Adults." *Morbidity and Mortality Weekly Report (MMWR)* 41, 17. Accessed online December 2008. http://www.cdc.gov/mmwr/preview/mmwrhtml/00018871.htm.

---

* Health officials in other countries may identify conditions not listed here that are common in their countries, for example, malaria in African nations.

that more effectively treat some of the diseases to which infected persons are more susceptible. As such, there is a much higher likelihood of persons infected with HIV to live more than ten years before being diagnosed with AIDS.

ARE HIV AND AIDS FOUND EVERYWHERE?

It is not uncommon to hear AIDS referred to as a modern epidemic. The word *epidemic* is defined by *Merriam-Webster's Dictionary* as "affecting or tending to affect a disproportionately large number of individuals within a population, community, or region at the same time" and as being "excessively present." This definition does fit the incidence of AIDS in the United States.

Almost one million people in the United States were diagnosed with AIDS during the first 25 years after AIDS was first reported in 1981 by the U.S. Centers for Disease Control and Prevention (CDC), based in Atlanta, Georgia. More than half a million Americans died of AIDS during that first quarter-century of the epidemic, and over 400,000 Americans are currently living with AIDS. As of 2006, more than 50,000 Americans a year had become HIV+ (CDC, 2008).

However, AIDS is not just an epidemic in the United States. It is a disease found in countries all over the world. In fact, many countries have much higher rates of AIDS and more people dying of the disease than the United States. That means AIDS is more accurately called a *pandemic,* meaning, as Merriam-Webster defines the term, "occurring over a wide geographic area and affecting an exceptionally high proportion of the population."

Worldwide in 2007, according to data compiled by the Joint United Nations Programme on HIV/AIDS (UNAIDS), an estimated 33 million people were living with HIV infection; almost 3 million people became infected with HIV that year and 2 million people died. Daily, over 6,800 people become infected with HIV and more than 5,700 die from AIDS (UNAIDS, 2007). The chapter in this book on "Prevalence" gives much more detail on numbers and rates of HIV and AIDS cases in the United States and globally.

WHERE AND WHEN DID AIDS BEGIN?

In the United States, the onset of the AIDS epidemic is commonly dated to 1981. That summer, the CDC issued a brief report describing five cases of *Pneumocystis* Pneumonia in young gay men in the Los Angeles,

California, area. The report in the June 5 edition of the CDC's *Morbidity and Mortality Weekly Report (MMWR)* was relatively brief. Including an editorial note and references, it was just over 1,000 words in length. The editorial note observed that

> *Pneumocystis* pneumonia in the United States is almost exclusively limited to severely immunosuppressed patients. The occurrence of pneumocystosis in these five previously healthy individuals without a clinically apparent underlying immunodeficiency is unusual. The fact that these patients were all homosexuals suggests an association between some aspect of a homosexual lifestyle or disease acquired through sexual contact and *Pneumocystis* pneumonia in this population . . . [the observations recorded in the report] suggest the possibility of a cellular-immune dysfunction related to a common exposure that predisposes individuals to opportunistic infections such as pneumocystosis and candidiasis. (CDC, 1981)

Within two months, the CDC had reports of 100 gay men with *Pneumocystis* pneumonia or a type of cancer know as Kaposi's Sarcoma. Like the specific type of pneumonia in the earlier report, this type of cancer was surprising in young, previously healthy men.

Following these reports, a team of CDC epidemiologists went to San Francisco and New York to learn more about these cases and to determine whether there was a new disease afoot. Epidemiology is the branch of medicine that focuses on the study of the causes, patterns, and control of disease. Epidemiologists investigate these things as a detective might investigate a crime. They gather data through testing biological samples, interviewing people about their behavior and activities, and following up on leads.

Although these medical investigators were not aware of it at the time, these early cases of AIDS reported by the CDC were not actually the first cases of AIDS anywhere. They were just the first cases systematically reported and recognized as exhibiting an unusual pattern of disease. Other cases that in retrospect would be identified as AIDS have subsequently been discovered as researchers have looked through medical records of individuals exhibiting the symptoms now known to be associated with AIDS and have tested biological samples from suspect cases. Such research has been able to establish Central African, European, Israeli, Canadian, and Haitian AIDS cases in the 1970s as well as a few cases in the United States that occurred before 1981 (Huminer and Silvio, 1988; Katner et al., 1987; Masur, 1982).

The earliest known case of HIV infection was discovered in a blood sample drawn in 1959 from a man in Kinshasa, Democratic Republic of Congo (formerly Zaire). That sample shows that HIV existed more than two decades before the first CDC report.

Although many theories about the origin of AIDS ranging from government conspiracies to aliens have been suggested, many researchers now generally agree that AIDS began somewhere in the Central African region. They believe that it likely developed from a simian virus that infected chimpanzees and somehow managed to cross over into humans, mutating into HIV perhaps in the 1930s. That could have happened when people ate the meat of, or were bitten by, the infected animals. Due to the geographic isolation of the area, the virus likely traveled out of the region slowly, eventually establishing itself in human hosts who spread the virus unaware of its existence.[1]

How Is HIV Transmitted?

Like all other epidemic and pandemic diseases throughout history, when AIDS was identified, there was a great amount of fear about how it could be transmitted. Particularly early in the AIDS crisis, before any AIDS medications were available and at which time AIDS was considered always fatal, fears were especially profound. Social stigmas such as the prevalence of HIV/AIDS among marginalized groups such as gay men and intravenous drug users compounded the fears and resulted in discrimination (see chapters 5 and 7). In some cases, people were so afraid that their behavior toward people who were infected with, or even suspected to have, HIV even became violent.

Researchers have now concluded that HIV is not an airborne virus like the influenza virus. That means someone cannot get infected with HIV, for example, by conversing with or sitting near someone in an airplane or theater who is HIV+. Fortunately, HIV is not a very robust virus when outside of the body. This means that it deteriorates fairly rapidly when not in an ideal environment like the body provides. It is neither able to replicate nor reproduce outside of the body, and any fluid that is infected with HIV that dries due to exposure to the outside environment effectively renders HIV dead. This is why the likelihood of contracting HIV from casual environmental contact is remote.

HIV is *not* transmitted by insects such as fleas (as was the case in the plagues that swept through the world during the medieval period), and it is not transmitted by mosquitoes (as is malaria or the West Nile Virus). Additionally, HIV is not transmitted by touching, hugging, or shaking hands with an infected person.

---

[1]See Stine, 2009, and Engel, 2006, for easily readable summaries of this research. Chapter 3 in this volume also addresses the research question of whether HIV is actually the cause of AIDS, as the mainstream medical community now holds to be the case.

HIV *is* transmitted through four body fluids: blood; semen; vaginal secretions; and breast milk. As such, prevention efforts have been, and continue to be, focused on limiting or eliminating the possibility of individuals transferring these fluids between one other. This is why there have been such well known public campaigns for safe (or *safer*) sexual practices, syringe exchange programs, and HIV testing for pregnant women; these campaigns have targeted the primary means of HIV transmission as a collective effort to reduce the likelihood of transmission.

Other unusual cases of HIV transmission have been documented, but upon investigation, all have involved some exchange of one of these infected body fluids (Stine, 2009). For example, in a rare case of transmission by deep kissing, both people had bleeding gum disease (CDC, 1997). In other rare cases in which transmission occurred from adult to child from HIV+ adults prechewing food for infants, the adults also had bleeding gum disease and fed teething children (Goldman, 2008).

How Does HIV Work?

Recall that HIV is the acronym for the **human immunodeficiency virus.** Notice that the final word in this sentence is *virus*; this is precisely what HIV is, a virus. Viruses are microscopic biological agents that are technically not considered to be living, as they do not meet the scientific requirements for what constitutes life (e.g., able to grow and reproduce, adapt to environmental conditions, etc.) They are only able to replicate and reproduce themselves through the use of other cells. Specifically, they attach (infect) themselves to a host cell and deliver their genetic material to the cell. They then hijack the cell's mechanisms for reproduction and use the cell to replicate many versions of themselves. Eventually, the cell becomes full of the replicated viruses and its structure begins to fail. The volume of replicated viruses in the cell causes the cell to burst, destroying the cell and releasing the replicated viruses to infect other cells. In this manner, the viruses spread to other cells replicating themselves, and in the process they destroy all of the cells used as replication centers.

HIV attaches to two types of white blood cells: T cells and CD4 cells. These cells are components of the human immune system, and their cellular health is vital to the health of the immune system. When HIV attaches to T-cells and uses them as hosts to create more copies of it, it destroys them in the process. Destruction of T-cells results in a critically impaired immune system; this, then is what leads to the condition known as AIDS.

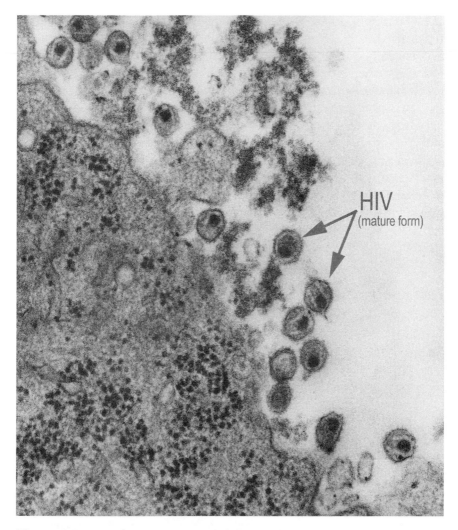

HIV
(mature form)

Figure 1.1 The Human Immunodeficiency Virus (HIV), a retrovirus, was identified in 1983 as the etiologic agent for the Acquired Immunodeficiency Syndrome (AIDS). AIDS is characterized by changes in the population of T-cell lymphocytes that play a key role in the immune defense system. In the infected individual, the virus causes a depletion of subpopulation of T-cells, called T-helper cells, which leaves these patients susceptible to opportunistic infections as well as certain malignancies. (Courtesy of Centers for Disease Control and Prevention)

So, HIV is simply the virus with which one gets infected. Preventing AIDS requires preventing HIV infection. This is why it is important to understand how HIV is contracted, how it spreads, who is most at risk, what kinds of prevention practices can be put in place, etc. If HIV is prevented, the development of AIDS is prevented.

As noted above, unlike infection from other viruses that result in changes in homeostasis in the body, infection with HIV does not immediately result in symptoms like chills, fever, aches, and pains, etc. Persons infected with HIV can live symptom free for many years; in fact, it is estimated that 25% of people infected with HIV are unaware of being infected. The only way to know if someone is infected is to get tested. This is why there has been an effort for the past 25 years for people to get tested for HIV. The chapters on medical research and on prevention and testing efforts provide more details on efforts to stop HIV/AIDS.

REFERENCES

Centers for Disease Control and Prevention (CDC). 1981. "*Pneumocystis* Pneumonia— Los Angeles." *Morbidity and Mortality Weekly Report (MMWR)* 30, 21: 1–3. Accessed online September 2008. http://www.cdc.gov/mmwr/Preview/mmwrhtml/june_5.htm.

———. 1982. "Update on Acquired Immune Deficiency Syndrome (AIDS)—United States." *Morbidity and Mortality Weekly Report (MMWR)* 31, 37: 507–508. Accessed online September 2008. http://www.cdc.gov/mmwr/preview/mmwrhtml/00001163.htm.

———. 1992. "1993 Revised Classification System for HIV Infection and Expanded Surveillance Case Definition for AIDS Among Adolescents and Adults." *Morbidity and Mortality Weekly Report (MMWR)* 41, 17. Accessed online September 2008. http://www.cdc.gov/mmwr/preview/mmwrhtml/00018871.htm.

———. 1997. "Transmission of HIV Possibly Associated with Exposure of Mucous Membrane to Contaminated Blood." *Morbidity and Mortality Weekly Report (MMWR)* 46, 27: 630–633. Accessed online September 2008. http://www.cdc.gov/mmwr/preview/mmwrhtml/00048364.htm.

———. 2008. "Cases of HIV Infection and AIDS in the United States and Dependent Areas, 2006." *HIV/AIDS Surveillance Report, 2006*. Vol. 18. Atlanta: US Department of Health and Human Services, CDC. Accessed online December 2008. http://www.cdc.gov/hiv/topics/surveillance/resources/reports/2006report/default.htm.

Engel, Jonathan. 2006. *The Epidemic: A Global History of AIDS*. New York: Smithsonian/Collins.

Goldman, Bonnie. 2008. "Three Cases of HIV Transmission to Infants through Food Pre-Chewed by HIV-Positive Caregivers." February 5. The Body Web Site. Accessed online December 2008. http://www.thebody.com/content/treat/art45178.html.

Huminer, David and Silvio D. Pitlik. 1988. "AIDS in the Pre-AIDS Era." *Canadian Medical Association Journal (CMAJ)*. 138, 5: 403.

Joint United Nations Programme on HIV/AIDS (UNAIDS) and World Health Organization (WHO). 2007. *AIDS Epidemic Update: December 2007*. Geneva, Switzerland: UNAIDS. Accessed online May 2009. http://data.unaids.org/pub/EPISlides/2007/2007_epiupdate_en.pdf.

Katner, H.P. and G.A. Pankey. 1987. "Evidence for a Euro-American Origin of Human Immunodeficiency Virus." *Journal of the National Medical Association*. 79, 10: 1068–1072.

Masur, Henry et al. 1982. "Opportunistic Infection in Previously Healthy Women: Initial Manifestations of a Community-Acquired Cellular Immunodeficiency." *Annals of Internal Medicine*. 97, 4: 533–539.

Stine, Gerald J. 2009. *AIDS Update 2008*. Boston: McGraw-Hill.

CHAPTER 2

HIV/AIDS Prevalence

In this chapter, we will look at:

- How HIV/AIDS data are collected
- What organizations collect these data
- What the data can tell us about the prevalence of HIV/AIDS in the United States and worldwide

Although many people have HIV/AIDS on their minds, it is sometimes hard to know exactly how many people are infected with HIV or are suffering from AIDS. Fears of HIV infection are not as rampant as they were when AIDS was first recognized and health professionals were uncertain about its transmission, but it is always helpful to get as complete a picture of the prevalence of the infection as possible.

WHAT IS PREVALENCE?

To begin, prevalence is defined as "The percentage of a population that is affected with a disease at a given time" (*Merriam-Webster,* 2007). In other words, prevalence can tell us how many people and what proportion of a population are affected by HIV/AIDS. Having this information is critical for current and future decision-making. Public health officials working to reduce and one day eradicate the spread of HIV/AIDS need accurate prevalence data to assist them in confronting the issues. Specifically, HIV/AIDS prevalence data assist in prevention, intervention, and education efforts.

How Are Prevalence Data Collected?

The two primary methods for collecting prevalence data are surveys and surveillance. Each method has limitations that will be discussed below.

Survey data-collection occurs by telephone, through the mail, in person, or on the Internet. Survey participants respond to a series of questions on the research topic, their answers are recorded, and their responses are analyzed. This is a popular and widely used method for collecting many types of data. Survey methods have several drawbacks, however, that can limit the accuracy of the data collected. These include: not being able to access all persons of interest (not everyone can be reached, some people refuse to participate, not everyone has a phone, or not everyone has Internet access); not getting complete responses (some people respond only to select questions or only fill out part of the questionnaire); and getting inaccurate information (some people forget times, dates, etc.; some do not disclose complete information; some lie).

The second method of prevalence data-collection is surveillance. Typically, one may think of surveillance as something law enforcement agents do (they put people *under* surveillance). With respect to gathering prevalence data on HIV/AIDS, however, it not this ominous. The CDC uses the definition from the *Merriam-Webster Dictionary* (2007), which defines surveillance as "to keep close watch over."

Indeed, this is what health professionals want to do with both HIV and AIDS. They want *to keep a close watch over* as many aspects of each respective condition as they can.

Governmental or local health agencies collect surveillance data. These data consist of information (test results, diagnoses, etc.) on people who present themselves for services (testing, treatment or both). Once recorded, they go to a data-collection clearinghouse for compilation and analysis. In the United States, the CDC serves this function; the World Health Organization (the WHO) provides this service for the rest of the world. The CDC primarily relies on surveillance methods to collect their HIV/AIDS data. The WHO uses surveillance and surveys. Like surveys, there are some challenges to data-collection with surveillance methods, too.

First, government and local health agencies in the United States are not necessarily required to report surveillance data to either the CDC or the WHO; they do so voluntarily. In the United States, virtually all state health agencies have been reporting AIDS data since 1981. In 1985, many began reporting data on HIV infection, too. Due to a number of different factors (lack of staff, lack of funding, not part of their mission), surveillance data are not reported on a regularly scheduled basis. As such, the CDC and the

WHO do the best they can to report the data that they have in a timely manner. The CDC and the WHO consistently work to improve surveillance data reporting from governmental and local agencies.

Surveillance data are from persons who present themselves for testing, through the screening of donated blood, death certificates, or medical treatment. In essence, surveillance data are *convenience* data; they represent data from a segment of the population, not *all* of the population. This results in a biased sample. Researchers correct for this by making prevalence *estimates* based on the data that they have. Inasmuch as researchers estimate the total number of people with HIV/AIDS who know they have HIV/AIDS, they also estimate the number of people who have HIV/AIDS who *do not* know that they do. For instance, the CDC reports that 24% to 27% of the estimated 1,039,000 to 1,185,000 people living with HIV/AIDS in the United States are unaware that they are HIV infected.

Despite these challenges, survey and surveillance methods provide the best available data for any person(s) interested in the prevalence of HIV/AIDS. We will now turn to the most recent surveillance data collected by the CDC on the prevalence of HIV/AIDS in the United States.

HIV/AIDS PREVALENCE IN THE UNITED STATES

As noted above, the central repository for HIV/AIDS surveillance data in the United States is the CDC. The CDC is an organization within the U.S. Department of Health and Human Services. Founded on July 1, 1946, as the Communicable Disease Center, its original mission was to fight the spread of malaria through exterminating mosquitoes; its first operating budget was less than $10 million.

Recently celebrating 60 years of service to the American public, its budget has grown to $8.8 billion, and its mission has broadened: "To promote health and quality of life by preventing and controlling disease, injury, and disability."

The CDC has two Divisions of HIV/AIDS Prevention (DHAP) that conduct prevention, surveillance, research, and evaluation activities. They also have a Global AIDS program that works internationally on HIV/AIDS issues.

The 2005 HIV/AIDS Surveillance report is the most recent prevalence report issued by the CDC. It is by far, the most comprehensive picture of the HIV/AIDS prevalence that we have. Due to some of the challenges noted in the previous section, these data are estimations, based on what is an 85% reporting rate (CDC, 2006). We will examine some of the most relevant findings below.

2007 HIV/AIDS Surveillance Report

Before we look at the data, we need to be clear on how the data are reported. Throughout the years, the CDC has clarified their understanding of the relationship between HIV infection and the development of AIDS. Continued research into these two conditions has resulted in changes in definitions, reporting standards, and reporting categories. Currently, there is a distinction made between HIV infection without an accompanying AIDS diagnosis, a diagnosis of HIV with a later diagnosis of AIDS, and a concurrent diagnosis of HIV and AIDS. Each of the tables that we will examine will note these differences in the titles of the respective tables.

Table 2.1 is a summary of HIV/AIDS data since 2003, broken down by age, gender, ethnicity, and transmission category. The total number of diagnosed cases in 2003 was 36,102 and 36,817 in 2006. Overall, the number of cases diagnosed has remained relatively stable. This suggests that prevention efforts have been successful in the past and continue to remain so. 2007 prevalence data have not been released, but it is unlikely that there will be a significant increase from 2006 numbers.

As you can see from the table, HIV/AIDS affects a wide range of ages from under 13 to over 65. There are more African Americans[1] affected by HIV/AIDS than any other group and the highest category of transmission is male-to-male sex.

Table 2.2 provides information on the amount of time from HIV infection to AIDS diagnosis based on two time frames: greater than or equal to 12 months after infection or less than 12 months after infection. Note that these data are for 2005. For the total number of people classified with HIV infection in 2005, 62% (22,197) received an AIDS diagnosis 12 months or longer after infection, and the remaining 38% (13,398) received an AIDS diagnosis less than 12 months after infection.

Age played a role in the time to AIDS diagnosis as we can see by observing that 88% of children under 13 received an AIDS diagnosis 12 months or longer after infection, and only 44% of people greater than or equal to 65 fell into that category. It is also interesting to note that 94% of children under the age of 13 who were infected by blood transfusion or another unidentified risk factor (the "Other" Transmission Category, received an AIDS diagnosis 12 months or longer after infection.

---

[1]There is no biological evidence for the existence of distinct races of people. Racial categories do exist, but they reflect human attempts at categorization, not analogs of categories that exist in nature. Current scientific evidence supports the notion that there is one race of humans with tremendous variation among the members (see Chapter 13 for more information on this). This is important to note when considering racial-ethnic categories and HIV/AIDS prevalence.

Table 2.1 Estimated numbers of cases of HIV/AIDS, by year of diagnosis and selected characteristics, 2003–2006. 33 states and 5 U.S. dependent areas with confidential name-based HIV infection reporting (Centers for Disease Control)

	Year of Diagnosis			
	2003	2004	2005	2006
Data for 33 states				
Age at diagnosis (yrs)				
<13	211	183	169	135
13–14	53	36	40	41
15–19	993	993	1,126	1,332
20–24	3,163	3,368	3,592	3,886
25–29	4,023	4,057	4,236	4,603
30–34	5,189	4,820	4,676	4,466
35–39	6,369	5,807	5,535	5,442
40–44	5,786	5,429	5,529	5,718
45–49	4,028	3,877	4,028	4,204
50–54	2,451	2,401	2,547	2,718
55–59≥	1,279	1,363	1,455	1,438
60–64	655	702	692	714
≥65	570	624	613	618
Race/ethnicity				
White, not Hispanic	10,033	10,181	10,528	10,758
Black, not Hispanic	17,668	16,718	16,629	17,356
Hispanic	6,355	6,010	6,217	6,481
Asian/Pacific Islander	338	339	373	397
American Indian/Alaska Native	179	171	182	166
Transmission category				
Male adult or adolescent				
Male-to-male sexual contact	15,409	15,880	16,833	17,465
Injection drug use	3,514	3,083	2,978	3,016
Male-to-male sexual contact and injection drug use	1,349	1,299	1,247	1,180
High-risk heterosexual contact[a]	4,269	3,959	3,871	4,152
Other[b]	125	110	107	114
Subtotal	24,666	24,331	25,036	25,928
Female adult or adolescent				
Injection drug use	2,027	1,856	1,720	1,712
High-risk heterosexual contact[a]	7,731	7,182	7,216	7,432
Other[b]	134	107	97	109
Subtotal	9,892	9,145	9,033	9,252

(Continued)

Table 2.1 *Continued*

	Year of Diagnosis			
	2003	**2004**	**2005**	**2006**
Child (<13 yrs at diagnosis)				
Perinatal	190	157	147	115
Other[c]	23	27	23	20
Subtotal	213	184	170	135
Subtotal for 33 states	34,770	33,659	34,239	35,314
Data for U.S. dependent areas	1,331	1,234	1,395	1,503
Total[d]	**36,102**	**34,894**	**35,634**	**36,817**

Note. These numbers do not represent reported case counts. Rather, these numbers are point estimates, which result from adjustments of reported case counts. The reported case counts have been adjusted for reporting delays and for redistribution of cases in persons initially reported without an identified risk factor, but not for incomplete reporting.

Data include persons with a diagnosis of HIV infection (not AIDS), a diagnosis of HIV infection and a later diagnosis of AIDS, or concurrent diagnoses of HIV infection and AIDS. See Technical Notes for the list of areas that have had laws or regulations requiring confidential name-based HIV infection reporting since at least 2003.

[a] Heterosexual contact with a person known to have, or to be at high risk for, HIV infection.

[b] Includes hemophilia, blood transfusion, perinatal exposure, and risk factor not reported or not identified.

[c] Includes hemophilia, blood transfusion, and risk factor not reported or not identified.

[d] Includes persons of unknown race or multiple races and persons of unknown sex. Because column totals were calculated independently of the values for the subpopulations, the values in each column may not sum to the column total.

Table 2.3 provides similar information to Table 2.1, but includes only those persons diagnosed with AIDS, and it also provides a cumulative total of reported AIDS cases since the epidemic began. As we can see, an estimated 1,014,797 persons have been diagnosed with AIDS since the epidemic began.

From Table 2.4, we can see the incidence of AIDS cases among children aged 13 and younger. This group accounts for less than 1% (9,144) of all AIDS cases since the epidemic began. Again, we see a higher incidence of AIDS diagnoses among children of African American descent. We can also see that in the majority of cases, HIV transmission was from mother to child. The good news here is that the incidence of AIDS cases among children aged 13 and younger has been in steady decline since 1992. This reflects the increase in knowledge about routes of transmission, comprehensive public awareness campaigns, and educational initiatives.

Tables 2.5 and 2.6 provide us another set of data. These tables permit us to see the rate of HIV/AIDS conditions among different populations. Population rates are better indicators of the prevalence of conditions

Table 2.2 Time to an AIDS diagnosis after a diagnosis of HIV infection, by selected characteristics, 2005—33 states and 5 U.S. dependent areas with confidential name-based HIV infection reporting (Centers for Disease Control)

	≥12 Months After Diagnosis of HIV Infection[a]		<12 Months After Diagnosis of HIV Infection[b]		Total
	No.	(%)[c]	No.	(%)[c]	No.
Data for 33 states					
Age at diagnosis (yrs)					
<13	148	88	21	12	169
13–14	22	54	18	46	40
15–19	912	81	215	19	1,126
20–24	2,874	80	714	20	3,589
25–29	3,077	73	1,157	27	4,234
30–34	3,016	65	1,655	35	4,671
35–39	3,353	61	2,176	39	5,530
40–44	3,181	58	2,338	42	5,519
45–49	2,145	53	1,874	47	4,019
50–54	1,307	51	1,239	49	2,546
55–59	725	50	728	50	1,453
60–64	316	46	376	54	692
≥65	266	44	346	56	612
Race/ethnicity					
White, not Hispanic	6,839	65	3,677	35	10,516
Black, not Hispanic	10,372	62	6,242	38	16,614
Hispanic	3,593	58	2,614	42	6,206
Asian/Pacific Islander	232	62	139	38	371
American Indian/ Alaska Native	110	61	72	39	182
Transmission category					
Male adult or adolescent					
Male-to-male sexual contact	10,917	65	5,902	35	16,819
Injection drug use	1,544	52	1,427	48	2,971
Male-to-male sexual contact and injection drug use	733	59	512	41	1,245
High-risk heterosexual contact[d]	2,091	54	1,773	46	3,864
Other[e]	45	42	61	58	107
Subtotal	15,331	61	9,675	39	25,006

(Continued)

Table 2.2 *Continued*

	≥12 Months After Diagnosis of HIV Infection[a]		<12 Months After Diagnosis of HIV Infection[b]		Total
	No.	(%)[c]	No.	(%)[c]	No.
Female adult or adolescent					
Injection drug use	1,056	62	660	38	1,716
High-risk heterosexual contact[d]	4,761	66	2,450	34	7,210
Other[e]	47	48	50	52	97
Subtotal	5,864	65	3,160	35	9,023
Child (<13 yrs at diagnosis)					
Perinatal	126	86	21	14	147
Other[f]	22	94	2	6	23
Subtotal	148	87	22	13	170
Subtotal for 33 states	21,343	62	12,857	38	34,200
Data for U.S. dependent areas	855	61	541	39	1,395
Total[g]	**22,197**	**62**	**13,398**	**38**	**35,595[h]**

Note. These numbers do not represent reported case counts. Rather, these numbers are point estimates, which result from adjustments of reported case counts. The reported case counts have been adjusted for reporting delays and for redistribution of cases in persons initially reported without an identified risk factor, but not for incomplete reporting.

See Technical Notes for the list of areas that have had laws or regulations requiring confidential name-based HIV infection reporting since at least 2003.

Data exclude 39 persons whose month of diagnosis of HIV infection is unknown.

[a] Includes persons in whom AIDS has not developed.

[b] Includes persons whose diagnoses of HIV infection and AIDS were made at the same time.

[c] Percentages represent proportions of the total number of diagnoses of HIV/AIDS made during 2005 for the corresponding group (see row entries).

[d] Heterosexual contact with a person known to have, or to be at high risk for, HIV infection.

[e] Includes hemophilia, blood transfusion, perinatal exposure, and risk factor not reported or not identified.

[f] Includes hemophilia, blood transfusion, and risk factor not reported or not identified.

[g] Because column totals were calculated independently of the values for the subpopulations, the values in each column may not sum to the column total.

[h] Includes 310 persons of unknown race or multiple races.

within specific groups than simple raw numbers of people. This is because different groups vary in size. For instance, the largest ethnic group in the United States is people identified as white or Anglo. By simply stating the raw numbers of people affected by HIV/AIDS, we do not know what percentage of that particular population is affected. By creating a constant (in this case, 100,000 people), we can compare the rate of

Table 2.3 Estimated numbers of AIDS cases, by year of diagnosis and selected characteristics, 2002–2006 and cumulative; United States and dependent areas (Centers for Disease Control)

	Year of Diagnosis					Cumulative[a]
	2002	2003	2004	2005	2006	
Data for 50 states and the District of Columbia						
Age at diagnosis (yrs)						
<13	106	70	53	53	38	9,156
13–14	62	74	70	66	73	1,078
15–19	316	302	334	410	401	5,626
20–24	1,399	1,568	1,624	1,675	1,669	36,225
25–29	3,137	3,059	3,196	3,110	3,423	117,099
30–34	5,701	5,521	5,144	4,668	4,349	197,530
35–39	8,217	8,017	7,072	6,479	6,402	213,573
40–44	7,404	7,626	7,703	7,378	7,298	170,531
45–49	5,358	5,617	5,498	5,727	5,628	107,207
50–54	3,271	3,364	3,491	3,527	3,687	59,907
55–59	1,607	1,693	1,836	1,861	2,071	32,190
60–64	872	864	913	872	955	17,303
>65	682	763	791	727	835	15,074
Race/ethnicity						
White, not Hispanic	11,233	10,948	11,066	10,676	10,929	394,024
Black, not Hispanic	19,246	19,512	18,909	18,081	17,960	409,982
Hispanic	6,712	7,102	6,771	6,823	6,907	161,505
Asian/Pacific Islander	425	450	444	450	519	7,951
American Indian/Alaska Native	177	176	182	170	155	3,345

(Continued)

Table 2.3 *Continued*

Transmission category	2002	2003	Year of Diagnosis 2004	2005	2006	Cumulative[a]
Male adult or adolescent						
Male-to-male sexual contact	15,709	16,078	16,054	15,711	16,001	465,965
Injection drug use	5,483	5,275	4,818	4,603	4,410	170,171
Male-to-male sexual contact and injection drug use	2,075	2,029	1,925	1,930	1,803	68,516
High-risk heterosexual contact[b]	4,547	4,471	4,506	4,306	4,558	65,241
Other[c]	253	226	228	237	217	13,893
Subtotal	28,067	28,079	27,532	26,787	26,989	783,786
Female adult or adolescent						
Injection drug use	2,897	2,836	2,810	2,586	2,385	74,718
High-risk heterosexual contact[b]	6,855	7,336	7,113	6,922	7,196	108,252
Other[c]	207	217	217	205	220	6,596
Subtotal	9,959	10,389	10,141	9,713	9,801	189,566
Child (<13 yrs at diagnosis)						
Perinatal	104	70	53	52	37	8,508
Other[d]	2	0	0	0	0	636
Subtotal	106	70	53	53	38	9,144

(Continued)

24

Table 2.3 *Continued*

	Year of Diagnosis					**Cumulative**[a]
	2002	**2003**	**2004**	**2005**	**2006**	
Region of residence						
Northeast	10,092	10,342	9,412	9,396	9,486	306,241
Midwest	4,125	4,226	4,089	4,371	4,164	101,479
South	17,198	17,630	18,225	16,894	17,104	374,800
West	6,718	6,339	6,000	5,891	6,074	199,978
Subtotal for 50 states and the						
District of Columbia	38,132	38,538	37,726	36,552	36,828	982,498
Data for U.S. dependent areas	1,058	1,060	921	955	833	31,217
Total[e]	**39,250**	**39,690**	**38,807**	**37,662**	**37,852**	**1,014,797**

Note. These numbers do not represent reported case counts. Rather, these numbers are point estimates, which result from adjustments of reported case counts. The reported case counts have been adjusted for reporting delays and for redistribution of cases in persons initially reported without an identified risk factor, but not for incomplete reporting.

[a] From the beginning of the epidemic through 2006.

[b] Heterosexual contact with a person known to have, or to be at high risk for, HIV infection.

[c] Includes hemophilia, blood transfusion, perinatal exposure, and risk factor not reported or not identified.

[d] Includes hemophilia, blood transfusion, and risk factor not reported or not identified.

[e] Includes persons of unknown race or multiple races and persons of unknown sex. Cumulative total includes 5,691 persons of unknown race or multiple races, 3 persons of unknown sex, 1,079 persons of unknown state of residence, and 3 persons who were residents of other areas. Because column totals were calculated independently of the values for the subpopulations, the values in each column may not sum to the column total.

Table 2.4 Estimated numbers of AIDS cases in children <13 years of age, by year of diagnosis and selected characteristics, 2002–2006 and cumulative; 50 states and the District of Columbia (Centers for Disease Control)

| | Year of Diagnosis | | | | | |
	2002	2003	2004	2005	2006	Cumulative[a]
Cumulativea Race/ethnicity						
White, not Hispanic	14	12	7	4	4	1,599
Black, not Hispanic	70	46	33	38	30	5,654
Hispanic	18	10	9	8	3	1,748
Asian/Pacific Islander	1	0	1	1	1	54
American Indian/Alaska Native	1	0	1	0	0	31
Transmission category						
Hemophilia/coagulation disorder	0	0	0	0	0	226
Mother with documented HIV infection						
or 1 of the following risk factors	104	70	53	52	37	8,508
Injection drug use	12	8	5	3	4	3,220
Sex with injection drug user	4	6	3	2	1	1,397
Sex with bisexual male	2	0	3	1	1	209
Sex with person with hemophilia	0	0	0	0	0	35
Sex with HIV-infected						
transfusion recipient	0	0	0	0	0	22

(Continued)

Table 2.4 Continued

	Year of Diagnosis					
	2002	2003	2004	2005	2006	Cumulative[a]
Sex with HIV-infected person, risk factor not specified	36	20	20	25	13	1,530
Receipt of blood transfusion, blood components, or tissue	2	1	0	0	0	144
Has HIV infection, risk factor not specified	47	34	21	21	17	1,951
Receipt of blood transfusion, blood components, or tissue	2	0	0	0	0	374
Other/risk factor not reported or identified	0	0	0	0	0	36
Total[b]	106	70	53	53	38	9,144

Note. These numbers do not represent reported case counts. Rather, these numbers are point estimates, which result from adjustments of reported case counts. The reported case counts have been adjusted for reporting delays and for redistribution of cases in persons initially reported without an identified risk factor, but not for incomplete reporting.

[a] From the beginning of the epidemic through 2006.

[b] Includes children of unknown race or multiple races. Cumulative total includes 58 children of unknown race or multiple races. Because column totals were calculated independently of the values for the subpopulations, the values in each column may not sum to the column total.

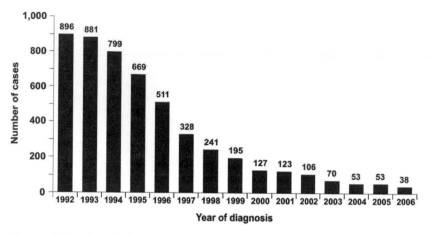

Figure 2.1   Estimated numbers of AIDS cases in children <13 years of age, by year of diagnosis, 1992–2006. Includes the 50 states and the District of Columbia. (Courtesy of Centers for Disease Control)

Note. These numbers do not represent reported case counts. Rather, these numbers are point estimates, which result from adjustments of reported case counts. The reported case counts have been adjusted for reporting delays, but not for incomplete reporting.

affected people within each group. This provides us with a better idea of the extent to which each group is affected. We already know from the previous tables that African Americans have the highest numbers of people affected, but how do those numbers compare to the numbers of affected people in other ethnic groups? We can see the extent to which each ethnic group is affected by looking at the data in Tables 2.5 and 2.6.

What do we see? That African Americans in general are affected by both HIV and AIDS at a much higher rate than any other ethnic category. Not surprising, both rates are higher for African American men, in each case more than twice as high as the rate for African American women. Persons identified as Asian/Pacific Islander have the lowest rates. We can also see that, in general, women have lower rates than men do.

Grouping prevalence data in this way allows prevention specialists and others to target certain groups for intervention. Knowing that African American men have the highest incidence rates is valuable information in this regard. By knowing this, advertising campaigns, outreach efforts, educational programming, etc., targeting African American men specifically can be undertaken. If, after engaging in intervention and prevention efforts, the rates for specific groups decrease, this can be taken as evidence of their efficacy.

Table 2.5 Estimated numbers of cases and rates (per 100,000 population) of AIDS, by race/ethnicity, age category, and sex, 2006; 50 states and the District of Columbia (Centers for Disease Control)

| | Adults or Adolescents | | | | | | Children (<13 yrs) | | Total[a] | |
| | Males | | Females | | Total[a] | | | | | |
Race/ethnicity	No.	Rate	No.	Rate	No.	Rate	No.	Rate	No.	Rate
White, not Hispanic	9,267	11.2	1,659	1.9	10,926	6.4	4	0.0	10,929	5.4
Black, not Hispanic	11,540	82.9	6,391	40.4	17,930	60.3	30	0.4	17,960	47.6
Hispanic	5,388	31.3	1,516	9.5	6,903	20.8	3	0.0	6,907	15.6
Asian/Pacific Islander	423	7.5	95	1.6	518	4.4	1	0.0	519	3.7
American Indian/Alaska Native	118	12.2	37	3.6	155	7.8	0	0.0	155	6.2
Total[b]	**26,989**	**22.4**	**9,801**	**7.8**	**36,790**	**14.9**	**38**	**0.1**	**36,828[c]**	**12.3**

Note. These numbers do not represent reported case counts. Rather, these numbers are point estimates, which result from adjustments of reported case counts. The reported case counts have been adjusted for reporting delays, but not for incomplete reporting. Data exclude cases in persons whose state or area of residence is unknown, as well as cases from U.S. dependent areas, for which census information about race and age categories is lacking.

[a] Because row totals were calculated independently of the values for the subpopulations, the values in each row may not sum to the row total.

[b] Includes person of unknown race or multiple races. Because column totals were calculated independently of the values for the subpopulations, the values in each column may not sum to the column total.

[c] Includes 358 persons of unknown race or multiple races.

Table 2.6 Estimated numbers of cases and rates (per 100,000 population) of HIV/AIDS, by race/ethnicity, age category, and sex, 2006—33 states with confidential name-based HIV infection reporting (Centers for Disease Control.)

| Race/ethnicity | Adults or Adolescents | | | | | | Children (<13 yrs) | | Total[a] | |
| | Males | | Females | | Total[a] | | | | | |
	No.	Rate	No.	Rate	No.	Rate	No.	Rate	No.	Rate
White, not Hispanic	9,078	16.7	1,664	2.9	10,742	9.6	16	0.1	10,758	8.2
Black, not Hispanic	11,230	119.1	6,033	56.2	17,263	85.6	93	1.7	17,356	67.7
Hispanic	5,058	50.9	1,400	15.1	6,458	33.7	23	0.4	6,481	25.5
Asian/Pacific Islander	318	13.5	79	3.2	397	8.2	0	0.0	397	6.7
American Indian/Alaska Native	129	17.7	35	4.6	164	11.0	2	0.6	166	8.8
Total[b]	25,928	33.8	9,252	11.5	35,180	22.4	135	0.4	35,314[c]	18.5

Note. These numbers do not represent reported case counts. Rather, these numbers are point estimates, which result from adjustments of reported case counts. The reported case counts have been adjusted for reporting delays, but not for incomplete reporting.

Data include persons with a diagnosis of HIV infection (not AIDS), a diagnosis of HIV infection and a later diagnosis of AIDS, or concurrent diagnoses of HIV infection and AIDS.

See Technical Notes for the list of areas that have had laws or regulations requiring confidential name-based HIV infection reporting since at least 2003.

[a] Because row totals were calculated independently of the values for the subpopulations, the values in each row may not sum to the row total.

[b] Includes persons of unknown race or multiple races. Because column totals were calculated independently of the values for the subpopulations, the values in each column may not sum to the column total.

[c] Includes 156 persons of unknown race or multiple races.

Another way to look at rates is by geographic location. It is interesting to note that rates vary by state, regardless of the population of the state. This tells us that there are apparent differences in population behavior that varies by location. For instance, the rate of diagnosed cases of AIDS in California (the most populous state in the union) is 207.2 per 100,000 people and in Washington, D.C. (one of the least populated areas in the union), it is virtually ten times that much; a rate of 2,016.2 per 100,000 people.

It is clear, by the data presented above that the HIV/AIDS pandemic is something that has had and continues to have a tragic presence in American life. As there is no vaccination against or cure for HIV/AIDS, the best method of prevention is through a sustained public awareness campaign that encourages the general public to refrain from, change, or eliminate certain behaviors; unfortunately, this is ongoing challenge.

GLOBAL PREVALENCE OF HIV/AIDS

For information on the prevalence of HIV/AIDS worldwide, we now turn to data collected by the World Health Organization (WHO). The WHO collects data from a number of different sources like the CDC and as such, is susceptible to the same limitations and restrictions.

World Health Organization

The World Health Organization was established by the United Nations in 1945. The UN wanted to create an organization that monitored and attended to global health issues. The WHO's constitution was officially recognized on April 1, 1948.

When it comes to the issue of HIV/AIDS, the WHO has five strategic directions (WHO, 2008):
1. Enabling people to know their HIV status through confidential HIV testing and counseling.
2. Maximizing the health sector's contribution to HIV prevention.
3. Accelerating the scale-up of HIV/AIDS treatment and care.
4. Strengthening and expanding health care systems.
5. Investing in strategic information to guide a more effective response.

The WHO is sort of the CDC for the world; they collect data, conduct research, make recommendations for prevention and intervention strategies, etc. They are based in Geneva, Switzerland, and are a valuable resource for information on medical needs and conditions throughout the globe.

The most recent report by the WHO and UNAIDS was released in 2008 and provides comprehensive data on HIV/AIDS worldwide (UNAIDS, 2008). We will look at several different trends and findings.

To begin, in 2007 there were an estimated 33 million HIV+ people in the world, with an annual total of 2.7 million new infections. It is also estimated that over 2 million people died of AIDS in 2007. Even though there has been a relatively stable number of people living with HIV since 2000, the number has been increasing each year.

Several regions of the world have been disproportionally affected by HIV/AIDS. One region in particular, Sub-Saharan Africa (the region of Africa that is located geographically south of the Saharan Desert) is one of these. This area alone accounted for 35% of global HIV infections and 38% of all AIDS deaths globally in 2007. Researchers also estimate that 67% of all persons living with HIV reside in Sub-Saharan Africa. This region of Africa remains home to the poorest population in the world. In all likelihood, with little opportunity for economic growth and development, this region of the world will remain beset by HIV/AIDS and other significant social issues for many years to come.

Not only are regions disproportionally affected by HIV/AIDS, so are different populations (we look at some of these in depth in later chapters). For instance, women account for 50% of all HIV positive people in the world and also account for almost 60% of infections in Sub-Saharan Africa. Similarly, children suffer disproportionately due to HIV/AIDS. Many lose parents and other significant people in their lives due to AIDS and become orphans. Perhaps even more tragically are those children who, through no fault of their own, become HIV infected. The WHO estimates that 2 million children are living with HIV, 370,000 children under the age of 15 became infected in 2007, and once again, almost 90% of those children live in Sub-Saharan Africa (UNAIDS, 2008).

Since 1990, the number of people living with HIV worldwide has increased from about 8 million to the current estimate of 33 million people. HIV prevalence since 1990 has also increased, however not at the same pace as the number of people living with HIV. Prevalence has increased from about 3 million people to just under 10 million (UNAIDS, 2008). In addition, as treatment options have improved and have increased in accessibility, the annual number of AIDS deaths has decreased in the last 10 years. Lastly, not including Sub-Saharan Africa, those populations that remain at high risk for HIV infection are intravenous drugs users, men who have sex with men, and those engaged in sex work (prostitution).

HIV/AIDS awareness, prevention, and treatment efforts over the last twenty years or so have improved greatly. The efficacy of these interventions varies depending upon the geographic region of the world and in some cases, the specific country. Like many other social conditions, the ability to effectively intervene in social problems is dependent upon the resources available, but unfortunately, resources are not distributed equally throughout the world. As such, some regions and countries are faced with much greater challenges in responding to the HIV/AIDS problem.

REFERENCES

Centers for Disease Control and Prevention. 2006. *HIV/AIDS Surveillance Report, 2005.* Vol. 17. Atlanta: U.S. Department of Health and Human Services, Centers for Disease Control and Prevention. CDC Web Site. Accessed online December 2008. http://www.cdc.gov/hiv/topics/surveillance/resources/reports/.

_____. 2007a. *AIDS Surveillance in the United States.* Retrieved May 2007, from http://www.cdc.gov/hiv/topics/surveillance/resources/software/apids/manual/section1.htm.

_____. 2007b. *Basic Statistics.* Retrieved May 2007, from http://www.cdc.gov/hiv/topics/surveillance/basic.htm#def.

Joint United Nations Programme on AIDS (UNAIDS). 2008. *2008 Report on the Global AIDS Epidemic.* Geneva, Switzerland: UNAIDS. Accessed online November 2008. http://www.unaids.org/en/KnowledgeCentre/HIVData/GlobalReport/2008/2008_Global_report.asp.

World Health Organization (WHO). 2008. *HIV/AIDS.* Accessed online November 2008. http://www.who.int/hiv/aboutdept/en/index.html.

CHAPTER 3

Medical Research on HIV/AIDS

In this chapter, we will look at

- The search for, and confirmation of, HIV as the cause of AIDS
- The development of pharmaceuticals to fight HIV
- Efforts toward developing an effective vaccine for HIV

When the CDC published its first reports in 1981 on the disease that would become known as AIDS, the medical community was baffled. The reports indicated complete breakdowns of the immune systems of young and previously apparently healthy individuals. The search for the cause of this immune dysfunction soon grew to include some of the most highly regarded researchers in the world and proved both challenging and contentious.

The knowledge gained from the unprecedented worldwide emphasis on HIV/AIDS research is proving useful in a myriad of other diseases as well. According to the National Institutes of Health's Office of AIDS Research (OAR) (2008), HIV/AIDS research has contributed to the development of

- Treatments for other viral and nonviral infections
- Better methods for preventing or combating opportunistic infections in those who have compromised immune systems, such as people undergoing cancer treatments or who have had an organ or bone marrow transplant
- Better understanding of the connections between viruses, the immune system, and cancers
- Advances in diagnosing and treating infectious diseases

- Important insights into the human immune system and into neurologic disease
- New approaches in designing and conducting drug trials
- Advances in the biotechnology sector
- Expanding the knowledge base for basic and clinical science
- Insights into human behavior that have improved public health knowledge and practice, health promotion, and disease prevention, and into better ways to research the social dimension of health and illness issues
- Progress in understanding newly emerging, or reemerging, infectious disease

Does HIV Cause AIDS?

The mainstream, scientific medical community now agrees that HIV is the virus that causes AIDS. In advance of the 13th International AIDS Conference held in Durban, South Africa, in 2000, more than 5,000 scientists and doctors, including Nobel Prize winners and directors of leading research institutes, signed the Durban Declaration affirming that HIV is the cause of AIDS. The signatories were published in the journal *Nature* (2000), which stated in an accompanying commentary that the "evidence that AIDS is caused by HIV-1 or HIV-2 is clear-cut, exhaustive, and unambiguous, meeting the highest standards of science."

The competition to discover the cause of AIDS was fierce and contentious, particularly between French scientists led by Dr. Luc Montaginer at the Institut Pasteur and those led by Dr. Robert Gallo at the U.S. National Institutes of Health. Controversy surrounding credit for the discovery of HIV made international headlines and grew to involve both governments. In 2008, Dr. Luc Montagnier and Francoise Barre-Sinoussi shared the Nobel Prize in Medicine for the discovery of HIV.

The Durban Declaration was in response to a controversy raging in South Africa over whether HIV causes AIDS. South African President Thabo Mbeki had aligned with a small group of HIV/AIDS dissidents and HIV/AIDS deniers. These are people who do not agree that HIV causes AIDS, or sometimes even that HIV or AIDS exists. Some favor conspiracy theories that blame pharmaceutical companies or government plots; others feel the science is inadequate; others find alternate explanations that better suit their personal experiences or beliefs ("Evidence," 2008).

In the United States, those who are well-known voices of dissent or denial include Christine Maggiore (2006). She is an HIV+ mother and former AIDS educator whose daughter died, according to the coroner, of

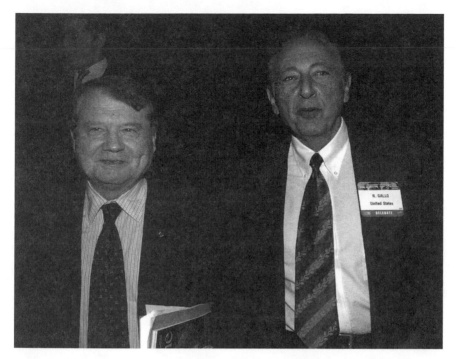

Figure 3.1   Leading AIDS researchers Dr. Luc Montagnier of France, left, and Dr. Robert Gallo of the United States leave after addressing the International AIDS Conference in Paris Monday, July 14, 2003. (AP Photo/Bob Edme)

AIDS-related causes. Dr. Peter Duesberg, a well-known virologist and cancer researcher, offers an opposing hypothesis that AIDS is caused by use of recreational drugs or even the drugs that treat HIV (Duesberg on AIDS, 2008). Dr. David Rasnick, a chemist who has published research on HIV medications and copublished a paper with Duesberg, has touted the risks of these therapies in South Africa. The Perth Group, a group of Australian researchers, argues that experts have not proven the "existence of a unique, exogenously acquired retrovirus, HIV" (the Perth Group, 2008).

Researchers look to four criteria that must be met to prove that an infectious agent causes a disease. These criteria are widely known as Koch's Postulates, named after the German scientist who proposed them in the late 1800s. The four postulates are

1. The causal agent (in this case, HIV) must be found in every person with the disease
2. The agent must be isolated from someone who has the disease and then grown in a pure culture

3. The agent must cause the disease when introduced into a healthy person
4. The agent must then be found in that infected person

Researchers who believe that HIV causes AIDS argue that each of these postulates have been met by solid science. Others disagree and argue that cases that do not fit into these postulates have been ignored, either purposely or overlooked due to poor scientific methodology.

In response to this contentious debate, the international HIV and AIDS charity Avert ("Evidence," 2008) summarizes, "There is no single scientific paper that proves HIV causes AIDS. Instead there are tens of thousands of papers containing a wide range of evidence that, taken together, make the case overwhelming. People should be encouraged to question scientific orthodoxy. However, the views of AIDS dissidents, which have been well known for many years and thoroughly debated in scientific journals, have failed to win support" (see "Evidence," 2008, and Stine, 2008 for detailed discussions).

DEVELOPING DRUGS TO TREAT HIV

Before HIV was isolated as the virus that causes AIDS, doctors were at a loss for effective ways to help their patients. They treated the opportunistic infections, but could do nothing about addressing the cause of AIDS, so AIDS was widely considered a death sentence. Desperate patients grasped at desperate measures.

AIDS HEALTH FRAUD

One aspect of treating HIV/AIDS, particularly early in the epidemic before the advent of any effective scientifically proven drug therapies or treatments to combat disease progression were developed, has been the problem of medical frauds. AIDS Health Fraud, defined by the U.S. Food and Drug Administration, is "the deceptive promotion, advertisement, distribution, or sale of articles represented as being effective to diagnose, prevent, cure, treat, or mitigate HIV/AIDS, or provide a beneficial effect on health, but which have not been scientifically proven safe and effective for such purposes. Such practices may be deliberate or done without adequate knowledge or understanding of the article." Fraud victims may be those with HIV/AIDS, their partners, family, or friends, as well as people who fear the risk of HIV infection.

As has been the case with other dread diseases in the past, those desperate for cures or succor have been targets for the intentionally deceptive to the well-intentioned but ineffective. The effects of AIDS health frauds range from benign to dangerous, even deadly. These interventions may interfere with legitimate treatments that have been scientifically shown to be effective in prolonging and improving the quality of life of those with AIDS, or they may delay such treatment. Additionally, such frauds may be expensive and not covered by insurance. Examples of AIDS fraud include individuals touting a wide variety of unapproved concoctions with no demonstrated medicinal value as treatment for AIDS, cancer, and other auto-immune diseases; sales of various bogus, unapproved, or medically useless HIV home test kits; and various unapproved and unproved electronic devices to kill HIV, cancer, and other diseases.

REFERENCE

AIDS Health Fraud Task Force Network. U.S. Food and Drug Administration. Office of Regulatory Affairs. Accessed online July 2008. http://www.fda.gov/ora/fed_state/dfsr_activities/aids_health_fraud_task_force.html.

Early researchers looking for a drug to combat HIV focused on experiments using known antiviral medications. These drugs generally did little to benefit patients; some had uncomfortable of even dangerous side effects, but they were the only hope many people with HIV and their loved ones had. When Ribavirin, an established drug used for viral respiratory disease, showed some potential in slowing the onset of AIDS, AIDS patients illegally imported it from Mexico before being able to obtain it for use against AIDS in the United States (Engel, 2006).

The first anti-HIV drug approved by the FDA as effective in fighting AIDS was azidothymidine, commonly known as AZT, and sold as Retrovir. It was approved for use by the FDA on March 19, 1987. Although the breakthrough in treatment was exciting, AZT therapy was cumbersome. It required some 12 pills per day, taken two at a time every four hours around the clock (Stine, 2008: 76). It was also extremely expensive: $3.00 per pill, or $8,000–$10,000 for a typical year's supply of medication. Public pressure eventually led to decreased costs. Even so, the drug was extremely profitable for the manufacturer, earning more than $300 million annually by 1994 (Engel, 2006: 129–131; Shah, 2006: 77–81). Even the World

Health Organization (WHO) in a 1994 meeting declined to endorse AZT for use around the globe for pregnant women due to costs and access issues, recommending a solution of "simpler and less costly" therapies be developed (Shah, 2006: 82–83). AZT also proved to have uncomfortable and even dangerous side effects as well (e.g., nausea, vomiting, headaches, fatigue, anemia, muscle pain and weakness, and neutropenia—a low white blood cell count that increases susceptibility to infection) to the extent that some patients stopped taking the drug.

Researchers raced to develop new drugs to fight HIV, yet the virus proved to be a formidable adversary. Researchers discovered that problems arose with so-called monotherapy—treating HIV with only one drug. When attacked with only one drug at a time, HIV mutated and became resistant to that drug. The resistant strains of HIV could then be passed on to others. In the United States, perhaps one-quarter of those infected with HIV who are "treatment-naive," meaning they have never received any HIV drugs, have a strain of HIV that is already resistant to some medications ("When the Drugs Don't Work," 2008).

As this problem became increasingly apparent to researchers and newer drugs became available, standard therapy for HIV starting in the mid-to-late 1990s became combination therapies that used various drugs together to combat HIV. Highly Active Anti-Retroviral Therapy, known by the acronym HAART, uses combinations of three or more drugs to reduce the chance of HIV drug resistance. Doctor David Ho of New York City's Aaron Diamond AIDS Research Center was recognized as *Time* magazine's Person of the Year for 1996 for his pioneering work on combination therapies (Chua-Eoan, 1996; Engel, 2006: 240–249). However, problems with side effects, patient adherence to difficult medication schedules (some requiring 30 pills to be taken throughout the day with varying dietary requirements), and high drug costs persisted (summarized in Engel, 2006). By 2008, over 25 different combinations of medications had been developed as "second line" therapies and even as "salvage" therapies to fight these drug resistant strains. One pill a day therapies—multidrug combination products—have also been developed to try to overcome some of the ongoing problems of resistance, side-effects, and cumbersome medication schedules. (See Diaz-Linares and Enid Vázquez, 2008; Gallant, 2008; and Stein, 2008 for detailed, but easily readable, discussions of drug therapies. Specific therapies for an HIV+ person should always be discussed with a knowledgeable medical professional).

Pharmaceutical development in the United States is a lengthy and expensive process involving a number of stages. In the early stages, the drug is developed and tested in a laboratory and on animals. If the drug is determined to be safe and produces promising results, it goes through a process requiring three more phases of testing on human volunteers. The next phases are called clinical trials. These phases take several years (for example, more than two years for the first phase and up to four for the third phase) and include larger numbers of people for testing at each stage of the process, ranging from 10 to 100 volunteers in Phase I, to several hundred in Phase II, to several thousand in Phase III. Researchers progressively build data on the safety, effectiveness, dosage, and any side effects. If the drug proves satisfactory, it may be licensed and become available for widespread use (FDA, n.d.; Kahn, 2005; Smith, 2003; NIAID, 2008a). Due to activism by HIV/AIDS advocacy groups, this process has actually been speeded up for HIV drugs.

At this writing, more than 30 antiretroviral drugs have been approved by the U.S. Food and Drug Administration to treat HIV (NIAID, 2008b). If positive outcomes occur when antiretroviral drugs are taken in the right combinations very soon after infection with HIV, some researchers are hopeful that long-term treatments may become unnecessary (Evans, 2008). Treatment with these drugs also appears to decrease the risk of non-AIDS related illnesses (e.g., cancers and cardiovascular, kidney, lung, and liver diseases) in HIV+ people with low CD4 cell counts (Moore et al., 2008). These drugs can, in many cases, suppress the virus so that it is "undetectable" in the body. However, none of these current drugs can "cure" HIV. If an HIV+ person stops taking their medication—even if they have reached a period in which the virus is at this "undetectable" level and the person feels no physical symptoms of illness—the virus

---

MAJOR CLASSIFICATIONS OF HIV DRUGS

1. Reverse Transcriptase (RT) Inhibitors

   AZT is in the nucleoside analog family of drugs that impact HIV through the reverse transcriptase enzyme in cells. A process called reverse transcription allows the genetic material in HIV contained in RNA, to be converted to DNA, the genetic material in human cells. This proviral DNA infects the healthy cells. Two types of RT Inhibitors interrupt this process. Nucleoside/nucleotide RT inhibitors (NRTIs), commonly called "nukes," block HIV from replicating in the cell by interrupting the RNA to DNA conversion process. Non-nucleoside RT inhibitors (NNRTIs), "non-nukes," prevent the conversion process by binding to the enzyme reverse transcriptase.

Combination HIV drug therapies frequently combine at least two nucleosides, considered the "backbone" of the treatment regimen, with one or more drugs from a different class. The idea behind this mixture is that drugs from different classes that work different ways will help to prevent resistance from occurring.

2. Protease Inhibitors (PIs)

The first protease inhibitor class anti-HIV drug, Saquinavir, was approved for use by the FDA on December 6, 1995. When HIV infects a CD4 cell, it uses that cell to make more HIV. It does this by making the cell produce proteins that it then uses to copy itself. The HIV proteins must be cut into smaller pieces by the enzyme protease for this process to work correctly, so that functioning copies of HIV can be made. Protease inhibitor drugs block the protease enzyme from doing this job, thereby blocking the ability of HIV to reproduce itself. Protease inhibitors were hailed as a breakthrough in the science of combating HIV/AIDS. Their approval made combination therapy possible.

3. Entry and Fusion Inhibitors

Entry and fusion inhibitors work as the name implies. Rather than trying to stop HIV after it has already infected a cell, these drugs work outside the cell. They interfere with HIV being able to enter, or fuse with, healthy CD4 cells in the first place. For HIV to infect a cell, the proteins on the surface of the HIV cell must bind with the receptor proteins on the surface of the CD4 cell. Entry and fusion inhibitors work by binding with either the HIV protein or the CD4 cell protein so that the HIV and healthy cell cannot bind, or fuse, with each other. They are used in combination drug therapies to fight HIV.

The first fusion inhibitor approved for use anywhere in the world was Fuzeon (enfuvirtide), which was approved by the FDA on March 15, 2003. The second, Selzentry (maraviroc), targeting a different protein, was approved several years later on August 6, 2007. These drugs may be especially useful to people who have become resistant to the other types of HIV drugs.

4. Integrase Inhibitors

After the process of reverse transcription is complete and the HIV RNA has been converted into DNA, the enzyme integrase integrates this viral DNA into the human DNA. Integrase inhibitors stop HIV from replicating by interrupting this integration process. Isentress (raltegravir) was the first drug in this class to be approved by the FDA in October 2007. Early reports showed encouraging clinical results without added side effects.

typically begins to increase again. This means drug treatment, as of this writing, is considered a lifelong state of affairs for most HIV+ individuals.

Due largely to advances in combination therapy research, the average life-expectancy and quality of life of those with HIV has increased significantly since the mid-1990s, from just under 7 years in the early 1990s to 24.2 years in the mid-2000s. However, the financial costs of these gains are high. The projected cost of lifetime treatment for HIV+ individuals is calculated at $618,900 per person, or approximately $2,100 per month (Schackman et al., 2006). Medications account for the majority of these costs.

Research on HIV therapies continues as researchers seek medications that work through different and hopefully more efficient mechanisms of action to fight HIV with fewer side effects. A database of HIV drugs currently under development in the United States is maintained by the Pharmaceutical Research and Manufacturers Association of America (http://www.phrma.org/). But not all new treatments will prove useful. For example, one novel treatment that attempted to speed up the HIV mutation rate to the point that it would basically mutate itself to death did not work (Dalton, 2008). Antiretroviral development remains central to fighting HIV/AIDS because vaccine development, another major focus of HIV/AIDS medical research, has been less promising.

IS IT POSSIBLE TO MAKE A VACCINE AGAINST HIV?

As defined by the National Institute of Allergy and Infectious Diseases (NIAID), a vaccine is, "a preparation that stimulates an immune response that can prevent an infection or create resistance to an infection." In simplest terms, a vaccine works by teaching "the immune system to recognize a specific harmful organism and fight off the disease when the body faces the real thing" (NIAID, 2008a). Medical researchers have developed effective vaccines against a number of deadly human viruses since the first vaccine against smallpox was developed in the 18th century (Jenner, 1798). Vaccines made the eradication of smallpox possible, as well as largely eradicating polio from most of the world. Vaccines are familiar and widely offered for other more common diseases, including measles and influenza.

Three types of vaccines might be useful in fighting HIV. According to Dr. Anthony S. Fauci, Director of the NIAID, a *preventive* vaccine that would protect people from becoming infected with HIV at all "remains the greatest hope for reversing the relentless spread of HIV" (Fauci, 2007). The International AIDS Vaccine Initiative estimates that if a preventive vaccine were even 70% effective that 28 million cases of HIV

Table 3.1 HIV medications—estimated cost per month

Class and Medication	Average Monthly Cost*
Protease Inhibitors (PIs)	
Aptivus	$1,072.80
Crixivan	$548.12
Invirase	$789.70
Kaletra	$794.99
Lexiva	$734.56
Norvir	$308.60
Prezista	$900.00
Reyataz	$927.14
Viracept	$726.40
Nucleoside Analog Reverse Transcriptase Inhibitors (NRTIs) or "Nukes"	
Combivir	$838.94
Emtriva	$368.93
Epivir	$386.93
Epzicom	$906.85
Retrovir	$432.88
Trizivir	$1,358.87
Truvada	$934.50
Videx and Videx EC	$367.93
Viread	$578.87
Zerit	$410.30
Ziagen	$519.92
Non-Nucleoside Reverse Transcriptase Inhibitors (NNRTIs) or "Non-Nukes"	
Intelence	$654.00
Rescriptor	$303.70
Sustiva	$531.04
Viramune	$463.85
Integrase Inhibitor	
Isentress	$1,012.50
Entry Inhibitors	
Fuzeon	$2,333.93
Selzentry	$1,044.00
Dual-Class Fixed Dose Combination	
Altripa	$1,465.54

* Costs may vary by dosage, by name brand drug or generic version (when available), and by where and in what quantities drugs are purchased. Also, a person may be taking more than one HIV medication at a time, further increasing their medication costs.

Diaz-Linares, Mariela, and Enid Vázquez. 2008. "12th Annual HIV Drug Guide." *The Journal of Test Positive Aware Network*. January/February. Accessed online November 2008. http://positively aware.com/2008/08_01/drug_guide.html.

could be averted between 2015 and 2030. Even a vaccine that was effective only half of the time could avert an estimated 17 million new cases of HIV infection during that time period (IAVI, 2008a). Fauci also acknowledges that even a *therapeutic* vaccine would have "enormous benefits." A therapeutic vaccine does not prevent infection; rather, it stimulates the immune system to "kick in to high gear," so to speak, to slow progression and reduce the likelihood of transmission to others. Another type of vaccine might be *perinatal.* This would be a vaccine administered to an HIV+ pregnant woman to prevent mother-to-child transmission of HIV.

Vaccines targeting HIV have been sought since early in the pandemic. When HIV was discovered in 1984, Margaret Heckler, Secretary of the Department of Health and Human Services, was hopeful for a vaccine within a few years (OTA, 1985). In 1997, President Bill Clinton called for a vaccine to be developed within 10 years. Controversial trials began in 1998 in the United States and in 1999 in Thailand for AIDSVAX, the first candidate HIV vaccine to reach Phase III clinical trials. The trial ended in 2003 when results showed it did not work ("HIV Vaccine Trial," 2003; Shah, 2006). In September 2007, large trials of another vaccine candidate conducted in several countries, the STEP and Phambili trials, were stopped early amid concerns that HIV infection rates were actually higher among those who received the vaccine than among the control group (Alcorn, 2008; Altman and Pollack, 2007). President Clinton's 10-year goal was not met; researchers around the world failed to produce an effective vaccine against HIV.

There are several reasons that developing a vaccine against HIV has proven to be so difficult. Some are scientific problems. HIV actually infects the very immune system cells that are supposed to fight viruses. HIV also has a high mutation rate, meaning that the virus is continually producing new strains that are different enough from the original infecting virus such that a vaccine targeting the original virus is no longer effective against it. Strains of HIV also differ by geographic region.

There are no documented cases of anyone "cured" of HIV that would help researchers better understand how recovery and immunity might work regarding HIV. Because they do not have animal models to help them study disease progression and predict how HIV vaccines might work, they have to rely on research on primates infected with a virus related to HIV, or ethically challenging and potentially dangerous human efficacy trials (NIAID, 2008a). Other impediments to HIV vaccine development are rooted in socioeconomic conditions, including poverty, lack of access to medical care, and lack of infrastructure, such as roads to readily transport medical supplies to rural areas or electricity or units for refrigeration.

So what would the ideal vaccine against HIV do? The IAVI (2008b) summarizes:

The ideal vaccine will protect immunized individuals against AIDS if they become exposed to any sub-type of HIV. The ideal vaccine will be effective worldwide, regardless of the ethnicity and nutritional and health status of the target population. The ideal vaccine will also protect against any route of HIV infection (vaginal, rectal, or oral sex; intravenous exposure; perinatal transmission); be inexpensive to manufacture; easy to transport and administer, even in remote areas of developing countries; stable under field conditions; and require few, if any, follow-up inoculations. Further, the ideal vaccine will have the capability for production in adequate quantities at an affordable cost, and have physical characteristics that make it amenable to worldwide distribution.

Some researchers have become discouraged about producing an HIV vaccine, but others are more confident that a vaccine can be developed. Organizations focusing on HIV vaccine issues include: the IAVI (http://www.iavi.org/); the Dale and Betty Bumpers Vaccine Research Center (VRC; http://www.vrc.nih.gov/), the HIV Vaccine Trials Network (http://www.hvtn.org/), and the Center for HIV/AIDS Vaccine Immunology (CHAVI; http://www.chavi.org/), all established by the NIAID; and the GAVI Alliance (http://www.gavialliance.org/), a partnership of a number of governments, researchers, corporate entities, the World Health Organization (WHO), the United Nations Children's Fund (UNICEF), the World Bank Group, and the Bill and Melinda Gates Foundation, among others.

REFERENCES

Acorn, Keith. 2008. "Study Shows How Vaccine May Have Increased Risk of HIV Infection." AIDSmap Web site. Accessed online November 2008. http://www.aidsmap.com/en/news/EF2D7C98-3FBF-4102-B05D-84503BB33C8D.asp.

Altman, Lawrence K., and Andrew Pollack. 2007. "In Tests, AIDS Vaccine Seemed to Increase Risk." *The New York Times*. November 8. Accessed online November 2008. http://www.nytimes.com/2007/11/08/health/08hiv.html?_r=1.

Chua-Eoan, Howard. 1996. "Dr. David Ho: Person of the Year Story." *Time*. Accessed online October 2008. http://www.time.com/time/subscriber/personoftheyear/archive/stories/1996.html.

Clavel, François, and Allan J. Hance. 2004. "HIV Drug Resistance." *New England Journal of Medicine*. 350, 10:1023–1035.

"Commentary: The Durban Declaration." 2000. *Nature*. July 6, 406: 15–16. Accessed online November 2008. http://www.nature.com/nature/journal/v406/n6791/full/406015a0.html.

Dalton, Paul. 2008. "Novel HIV Therapy Suffers Stunning Setback." The Body Web Site. June 12. Accessed online October 2008. http://www.thebody.com/content/treat/art47195.html.

Diaz-Linares, Mariela, and Enid Vázquez. 2008. "12th Annual HIV Drug Guide." *The Journal of Test Positive Aware Network*. January/February. Accessed online November 2008. http://positivelyaware.com/2008/08_01/drug_guide.html.

"Duesberg on AIDS." 2008. Peter Duesberg Web Site. Accessed online November 2008. http://www.duesberg.com/.

Engel, Jonathan. 2006. *The Epidemic: A Global History of AIDS*. New York: Smithsonian Books/Collins.

Evans, David. 2008. "A 'Functional' Cure for HIV." POZ Magazine Web Site. Accessed online October 2008. http://www.poz.com/articles/hiv_cure_fauci_401_15255.shtml.

"Evidence that HIV Causes AIDS." 2008. November 11. Avert Web site. Accessed online November 2008. http://www.avert.org/evidence.htm.

Fauci, Anthony S. 2007. "25 Years of HIV/AIDS Science: Reaching the Poor with Research Advances." *Cell*. 1331, 3: 429–432. Accessed online September 2008. http://www3.niaid.nih.gov/relatedArticles/cell131_31.htm.

Food and Drug Administration (FDA). No date. "The FDA's Drug Review Process: Ensuring Drugs Are Safe and Effective." FDA Web site. Accessed online September 2008. http://www.fda.gov/fdac/special/testtubetopatient/drugreview.html.

Gallant, Joel. 2008. "HIV Drug Guide Introduction." *The Journal of Test Positive Aware Network*. January/February. Accessed online November 2008. http://positivelyaware.com/2008/08_01/drug_guide_introduction.html.

Heckler, Margaret M. Secretary, U.S. Department of Health and Human Services, Washington DC, Statement Regarding AIDS, April 23, 1984.

"HIV Vaccine Trial Ends in Failure." 2003. *BBC News*. November 12. BBC News Web site. Accessed online November 2008. http://news.bbc.co.uk/1/hi/health/3265089.stm.

International AIDS Vaccine Initiative (IAVI). 2008a. "The Potential Impact of an AIDS Vaccine." IAVI Web site. Accessed online October 2008. http://www.iavi.org/viewpage.cfm?aid=1367.

_____. 2008b. "The Urgent Global Need for an AIDS Vaccine." IAVI Web site. Accessed online October 2008. http://www.iavi.org/viewfile.cfm?fid=1144.

Jenner, E. 1798. *An Inquiry into the Causes and Effects of Variolae Vaccinae, a Disease Discovered in Some Western Counties of England*. London: Sampson Low.

Kahn, Patricia, ed. 2005. *AIDS Vaccine Handbook: Global Perspectives*. New York: AIDS Vaccine Advisory Coalition.

Maggiore, Christine. 2006. *What If Everything You Thought You Knew About AIDS Was Wrong?* Van Nuys, CA: American Foundation for AIDS Alternative.

Markel, Howard. 2004. "'Who's On First?'—Medical Discoveries and Scientific Priority." *New England Journal of Medicine*. December 30: 2792–2793.

Moore, Richard D., Kelly A. Gebo, Gregory M. Lucas, and Jeanne C. Keruly. 2008. "Rate of Comorbidities Not Related to HIV Infection or AIDS among HIV-Infected Patients, by CD4 Cell Count and HAART Use Status." *Clinical Infectious Diseases*. 47, 8: 1102–1104.

National Institute of Allergy and Infectious Diseases (NIAID). 2008a. "Challenges in Designing HIV Vaccines." NIAID Web Site. Accessed October 2008. http://www3.niaid .nih.gov/topics/HIVAIDS/Understanding/Vaccines/vaccineChallenges.htm.

National Institute of Allergy and Infectious Diseases (NIAID). 2008b. "Treatment of HIV Infection." NIAID Web Site. Accessed October 2008. http://www3.niaid.nih.gov/NR/ exeres/A01539FA-7571-48C4-8A76-C526D5F7EFE9.htm.

Office of AIDS Research (OAR). 2008. "Research on AIDS Benefits Efforts against Other Diseases." Bethesda, MD: National Institutes of Health. Accessed online October 2008. http://www.oar.nih.gov/hivaids/crossoverbenefits.asp.

Office of Technology Assessment (OTA). 1985. *Review of the Public Health Service's Response to AIDS*. OTA-TM-H-24. February. Washington, DC: U.S. Congress. Accessed online November 2008. http://www.princeton.edu/~ota/disk2/1985/8523/8523.PDF.

"The Perth Group HIV/AIDS Debate." 2008. The Perth Group Web site. http://www .theperthgroup.com/.

Schackman, Bruce R., Kelly A. Gebo, Rochelle P. Walensky, Elena Losina, Tammy Muccio, Paul E. Sax, Milton C. Weinstein, George R. Seage III, Richard D. Moore, and Kenneth A. Freedberg. 2006. "The Lifetime Cost of Current Human Immunodeficiency Virus Care in the United States." *Medical Care*. 44, 11: 990–997.

Shah, Sonia. 2006. *The Body Hunters: Testing New Drugs on the World's Poorest Patients*. New York: New Press.

Smith, Kendall A. 2003. "The HIV Vaccine Saga." *Medical Immunology*. 2, 1. Accessed online October 2008. http://www.medimmunol.com/content/2/1/1.

"When the Drugs Don't Work: HIV is Growing More Resistant to Treatment." 2008. *Financial Times*. August 1: 7.

CHAPTER 4

Prevention, Education, and Testing

In this chapter, we will look at

- An overview of the focus of programs aimed at HIV prevention and education
- The growing trend in using media and celebrities in HIV/AIDS education and prevention programs
- Testing for HIV infection as a crucial feature of prevention efforts

When diseases are transmitted through airborne viruses or carried by insects or transmitted in ways that people do not understand, spread of the disease is difficult to prevent and stop. People risk infection by casual contact or even by being in close proximity with those who are infected. However, HIV is different. It is not transmitted casually; by avoiding contact with infected blood, semen, vaginal secretions, or breast milk, transmission of the virus and infection is preventable. As many commentators have noted, until doctors find a medical way to cure HIV, prevention *is* the cure. Educational efforts that give people the tools they need for prevention along with testing that allows people to know their HIV status and safeguard themselves and others are crucial aspects of arresting the HIV/AIDS pandemic. Difficulties arise from this deceptively simple sounding solution because even educated people do not always engage in safe behaviors, and societal factors can impact educational and prevention efforts in detrimental, as well as productive, ways.

PREVENTION AND EDUCATION PROGRAMS

The first HIV prevention efforts in the United States were grassroots efforts undertaken in 1982 by gay advocacy groups in San Francisco and New York who were reacting to the crisis afflicting members of those gay communities. With little data available at the time, they primarily focused on raising awareness; providing basic information about symptoms, probable modes of transmission, and risk-reduction; and quelling fears (CDC, 2006).

Government-instituted prevention-oriented programs took various forms throughout the 1980s. Early efforts primarily targeted groups considered at high-risk for contracting HIV, youth, racial and ethnic minority populations, and health-care workers. Program leaders were also concerned about perinatal transmission. An unprecedented educational effort by the federal government to reach mainstream America was an eight-page brochure, "America Responds to AIDS," that was mailed to more than one million American households in 1988. Overseen by Surgeon General C. Everett Koop, the brochure and content were created amidst controversy in President Ronald Reagan's conservative administration, which had delayed production for over a year. It revised Koop's initial "unusually explicit" report that had encouraged "frank, open discussions" between parents and children about AIDS, as well as public education about facts and risk factors. It also predicted the increases in heterosexual transmission emerging later in the epidemic (Boffey, 1986).

Political conservatism has also been central to one of the most contentious issues in HIV prevention in the United States—sex education in schools. The Bush administration pressed an abstinence-based sex education curriculum rather than a more comprehensive curriculum covering information on topics such as condom use and safer sex. However, research shows that abstinence-only sex education programs do not best impact risk of HIV; education initiatives that are more broadly focused are more effective (Alford, 2008; SIECUS, 2007; Underhill, Montgomery, and Operario, 2007). Abstinence-only education programs also do not reflect what most Americans favor. A Kaiser Family Foundation poll (2006) found that only 10% of Americans thought HIV prevention programs that focus mainly on abstinence more closely fit their beliefs than those focusing mainly on safer sex and condom use (13%) or combined approaches including abstinence, monogamous sexual relationships, and condom use (75%).

In community-based and clinic settings, some characteristics of programs that have shown promise are programs that are culturally based to reach various populations; use various cognitive behavioral theories; address the social factors such as abuse and exploitative sexual practices

Table 4.1   Officially recognized AIDS days

HIV/AIDS Awareness Days	
Event	**Date**
National Black HIV/AIDS Awareness Day	February 7
National Women & Girls HIV/AIDS Awareness Day	March 10
National Native HIV/AIDS Awareness Day	March 20
HIV Vaccine Awareness Day	May 18
National Asian & Pacific Islander HIV/AIDS Awareness Day	May 19
Caribbean American HIV/AIDS Awareness Day	June 8
National HIV Testing Day	June 27
National Latino AIDS Awareness Day	October 15
World AIDS Day	December 1

"HIV/AIDS Awareness Days." U.S. Department of Health and Human Services. Accessed online September 2008. http://www.hhs.gov/aidsawarenessdays/.

that lead to increased transmission of HIV; address HIV-related stigma; teach young women skills necessary to use condoms; emphasize gender empowerment, partner negotiation skills, healthy relationships, and reducing the number of sexual partners; and may also incorporate the use of support groups (e.g., Alford, 2008; DiClemente and Crosby, 2006). A variety of HIV/AIDS awareness days also call attention to the issue. (See Table 4.1 for awareness days officially recognized in the United States.)

While community and government efforts did increase basic knowledge about HIV transmission and prevention, reduce some risk behavior, and decrease negative attitudes toward persons living with HIV/AIDS, they were much less successful in getting some in high-risk populations to change their behavior (CDC, 2006). In 2003, amidst mounting concerns about increasing rates of HIV and in light of the availability of rapid HIV testing technology (discussed below), CDC prevention emphases shifted to four key strategies:

1. Making HIV testing a routine part of medical care
2. Implementing new models for diagnosing HIV infections outside medical settings (e.g., by AIDS Service Organizations conducting testing at community events)
3. Preventing new infections by working with persons diagnosed with HIV and their partners to change risky behavior and to maintain that change
4. To further decrease perinatal HIV transmission through routine HIV testing of all pregnant women (CDC, 2003)

MICROBICIDES

Microbicides, as the name suggests, are designed to kill microbes (such as viruses) that could cause infection or illness. To protect against transmission of HIV and other sexually transmitted infections, these would be creams, gels, films, pills, or suppositories that would be inserted into the vagina or rectum. They might be used alone or in combination with other barriers such as condoms. According to the Alliance for Microbicide Develepment, at the end of 2008, 60 microbicides were in some stage of the development "pipeline" (AMD, 2008).

Particularly in developing countries, microbicides would offer an alternative to condom use. Their availability "would greatly empower women to protect themselves and their partners. Unlike male or female condoms, microbicides are a potential preventive option that women can easily control and do not require the cooperation, consent, or even knowledge of the partner" (WHO, 2008). Even a microbicide with only low effectiveness could prevent an estimated 6 million cases of HIV over three years at a cost savings of over $3 billion dollars (WHO, 2008).

REFERENCES

Alliance for Microbicide Development (AMD). 2008. "Microbicide Pipeline." AMD Web site. Accessed online December 2008. http://www.microbicide.org/cs/microbicide_pipeline.
World Health Organization (WHO). 2008. "Microbicides." WHO Web site. Accessed online December 2008. http://www.who.int/hiv/topics/microbicides/microbicides/en/.

Around the globe, prevention and education programs take diverse forms, and they should be culturally specific and appropriate to be effective. According to the Global HIV Prevention Working Group (2007), an international group of more than 50 experts in HIV/AIDS, the key to global prevention is "the right interventions focused on the right people at the right scale." Their report identifies essentials to which people worldwide must have access for prevention to occur on a scale that can make a difference in stemming the pandemic. Access to each is especially problematic in poorer countries. (See the sidebar on Microbicides for one possible future intervention that may especially benefit poorer areas of the world.) These essentials are

- Condoms—They are often unavailable and are used in less than 10% of risky acts worldwide.
- HIV testing—People should be able to know their status; for example, less than 12% of those in sub-Saharan Africa know their status.
- Treatment for sexually transmitted infections (STIs)—STIs increase the likelihood of HIV transmission.
- Prevention of mother-to-child transmission—Antiretroviral medications that can cut the mother-to-child transmission rate by 50% are available to only 11% of women in some poorer countries.
- Focus on high-risk populations—High-risk populations include men who have sex with men, sex workers, and intravenous drug users.
- Prevention in health care settings—Product blood screening and sterile needles and equipment are often unavailable.

PREVENTION AND EDUCATION CAMPAIGNS USING MEDIA

Media technology is increasingly utilized in public education campaigns, including those for HIV/AIDS awareness and prevention ("The Digital Opportunity," 2007) and is continuing to expand globally, reaching more consumers (especially youth) than ever before. More people have access to media technology than at any other time in history, giving the media an extraordinarily wide reach for disseminating information.

Tied to these trends are entertainment-education communication strategies that purposefully combine entertainment and educational messages to enact or reinforce changes in attitudes, beliefs, values, and behavior. Entertainment-education communication strategies were pioneered by Miguel Sabido of Mexico's Televisa network. The Peruvian *Simplemente Maria*, a serial that featured a young woman dealing with several issues, including HIV, demonstrated the effectiveness of this approach that is now used worldwide (Brown and Singhal, 1999).

In 2004, United Nations Secretary General Kofi Annan publicly called for increasing media participation in HIV/AIDS education and prevention efforts. The result was the Global Media AIDS Initiative. Public service messages on HIV/AIDS have aired around the world including the United States, India, China, Russia, and Africa. Collaborations between the Asia-Pacific Broadcasting Union (ABU), an association of more than 150 radio and TV broadcasters, MTV International, the Kaiser Family Foundation, and several United Nations agencies have resulted in television programming initiatives to raise awareness and encourage behavior change ("ABU," 2005). As one example, the Coca Cola Africa

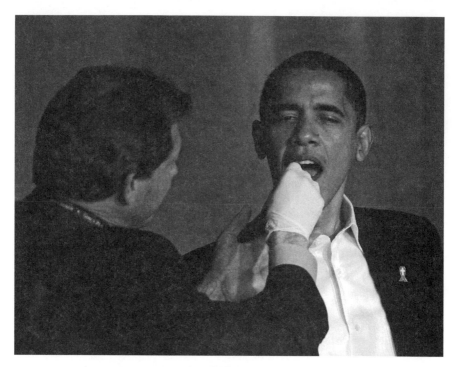

Figure 4.1 President Barack Obama, then a senator from Illinois, takes an HIV test during his appearance at the 2006 Global Summit on AIDS and the Church at the Saddleback Church in Lake Forest, California, in December 2006. (AP Photo/Damian Dovarganes.)

Foundation has been among the supporters of *SIDA dans la Cité (SDLC)*, or *AIDS in the City*, an educational television drama series aired in several western and central African nations. "Global collaborations among government, public health organizations and media companies have turned the entertainment industries on several continents into one of the most powerful public health communications tools of the 21st century" (Sternberg, 2006).

But do these efforts that leverage media outlets make a difference? Research shows that they can. In addition to the success of *Simplemente Maria*, research has also found safer sex behavioral changes among *SDLC* viewers (e.g., Shapiro, Meekers, and Tambashe, 2003). A South Africa television serial that positively portrays characters living with HIV, *Tsha Tsha*, supported by the U.S. President's Emergency Plan for AIDS Relief through the USAID, also shows results. Researchers found that after viewing a season of the show, viewers (as compared with nonviewers) were more likely to have positive attitudes and increased knowledge about HIV/AIDS, including HIV/AIDS-related stigma; an increased sense of responsibility for others' well-being; and to practice HIV preventive behaviors, including taking an HIV test. Overall, viewers saw the series as "realistic, captivating, entertaining, and educational" (Health Communication Partnership, 2006). Research on Kenyan military personnel based on the film *Red Card: Sammy's Final Match* (2005), which featured a Kenyan celebrity soccer player, also found positive behavioral changes (Brown, Fraser, and Kiruswa, 2004). Learning whether these types of behavioral changes are long-term across years or only of shorter duration remains an ongoing research goal.

Testing

Testing is central to CDC HIV prevention strategies (CDC, 2003, 2007). Various public figures around the world, including President Obama (as shown in the accompanying photograph) have been publicly tested to emphasize the importance of knowing one's HIV status. It is important for those who are HIV+ to know their status so that they can make informed decisions regarding treatment and health decisions. Those who are HIV+ receive additional tests from their health care provider to help guide treatment decisions, such as when to start taking HIV medications and how well those medications are working. Additionally, once they know they are infected, many HIV+ people take precautions to protect their sex or needle-sharing partners from transmission (CDC, 2008a; Holtgrave and Anderson, 2004). (See the CDC statement in Appendix B on "Deciding If and When To Be Tested.")

According to CDC data, between 16 and 22 million people are tested for HIV in the United States each year. However, one-quarter of the estimated one million persons living with HIV in the United States are unaware that they are infected. Also, many people have been infected for years before they are tested. Almost 40% of people who were first diagnosed with HIV in 2005 developed AIDS within a year of their diagnosis (CDC, 2008b). Because AIDS generally takes years to develop (perhaps even a decade or more), these people had been HIV+ for a long period of time.

In the United States, as in some other countries, issues surrounding HIV testing have long been contentious. Various interest groups, including politicians, physician's organizations, gay rights advocates, attorneys, and others, have contentiously debated—sometimes shifting positions— whether testing should be mandatory (and if so, for whom) and whether positive results should be reported by name to authorities or to sexual partners. Proponents of these measures argue that they are necessary to guard the public health; opponents argue the threats to confidentiality and civil liberties outweigh any potential benefits. At this writing, requirements vary by state.

Rather than looking for HIV itself, most HIV tests look for the antibodies (specific proteins) that the body develops in reaction to HIV. The most common screening test that looks for HIV antibodies is the Enzyme-Linked Immunosorbent Assay (ELISA). These tests commonly use blood samples drawn from a vein. Properly conducted ELISA blood tests are considered 99.9% accurate. That means that only one person in every thousand will receive an incorrect result from the test, either a false positive or false negative. Other ELISA tests have been developed that use oral fluid from the gums collected by a special apparatus. Yet another test analyzes a subject's urine. A positive result on an ELISA test must be confirmed with a follow-up test such as the Western Blot (a more specific antigen test) before a diagnosis of HIV is made.

The antibodies that these tests look for take from two to eight weeks or even longer to develop in people who become infected with HIV. The average is 25 days. Ninety-seven percent of people who contract HIV will develop antibodies within three months of becoming infected. If subjects take this HIV antibody test during this "window period" between infection and development of detectable antibody levels, their test results may appear negative for the virus; however, they can still transmit the virus to others. To account for this window, the CDC recommends that those who test negative within the first three months after an exposure or possible exposure to HIV should be tested again after six months to be sure the results are accurate.

HIV testing is continually being refined and improved. Tests are also available that look for HIV genetic material. These antigen tests can detect HIV infection before antibodies develop by looking for the p24 protein, the HIV protein that actually causes the body to develop antibodies. This is used for blood supply screening in the United States, and it can be used to screen individuals as well. Polymerase Chain Reaction (PCR) testing looks for genetic material of HIV itself in the viral DNA or RNA. This process is also used to detect HIV in blood donors during this window period. Additionally, this procedure is used to test newborns of HIV positive mothers and to assess viral load (i.e., the level of virus in the blood), which can show how well treatments are working. (See Appendix B for a CDC statement on the safety of the blood supply in the United States.)

Rapid tests have been developed that test for HIV-antibodies in oral fluid, urine, and finger-prick blood. Rather than waiting days or weeks for laboratory results, rapid tests provide reliable results in approximately 20 minutes (Greenwald et al., 2006). These rapid-result tests are important not only to lessen the anxiety that waiting on results can cause, but also because research shows that between 12.5% and 30% of those tested (depending on testing site) who have to return to the testing site to get their results do not return (Greenwald, 2006). Confirmation tests conducted by a laboratory are required when rapid tests show a positive result and involve a longer wait.

In 1996, a home collection HIV test system was approved by the U.S. Food and Drug Administration (FDA). Until then, people had to get their HIV tests in professional health care settings. The FDA had long opposed home testing because of concerns that those tested would not receive adequate counseling, a concern that had to be addressed to the satisfaction of FDA decision-makers before approval. More than a decade later, still only one home collection test system (i.e., the "Home Access HIV-1 Test System" or the "Home Access Express HIV-1 Test System" manufactured by Home Access Health Corporation) is approved by the FDA for legal marketing in the United States. It is available without a prescription at pharmacies and sold on the Internet; however, other unapproved kits are sold on the Internet as well. This home collection test system allows the user to take blood samples at home by a finger prick and get anonymous results after sending the blood in for laboratory analysis. (There is no home test kit that allows the user to interpret test results themselves.) If the results are positive, a second test will be performed for confirmation. The accuracy rate of these approved home test systems is comparable to tests offered in professional settings. Counseling and even medical referrals are provided for those who test HIV+; counseling on how not to contract HIV is provided for those who test negative for the virus (FDA, 2008).

REFERENCES

"ABU Unveils HIV/AIDS Initiatives." 2005. WorldScreen.com Web site. November 30. Accessed online October 2008. http://www.worldscreen.com/newscurrent.php?filename=abu1130.htm.

Alford, S. 2008. *Science and Success, Second Edition: Sex Education and Other Programs That Work to Prevent Teen Pregnancy, HIV & Sexually Transmitted Infections.* Washington DC: Advocates for Youth. Accessed online September 2008. http://www.advocatesforyouth.org/programsthatwork/intro.htm.

Boffey, Philip M. 1986. "Surgeon General Urges Frank Talk to Young on AIDS." *The New York Times.* October 23. Accessed online December 2008. http://query.nytimes.com/gst/fullpage.html?res=9A0DE4DC1F38F930A15753C1A960948260&sec=health&spon=&pagewanted=1.

Branson, Bernard M., H. Hunter Handsfield, Margaret A. Lampe, Robert S. Janssen, Allan W. Taylor, Sheryl B. Lyss, and Jill E. Clark. 2006. "Revised Recommendations for HIV Testing of Adults, Adolescents, and Pregnant Women in Health-Care Settings." *Morbidity and Mortality Weekly Report (MMWR).* September 22. 55, RR14:1–17. Centers for Disease Control and Prevention (CDC) Web site. Accessed online December 2008. http://www.cdc.gov/mmwr/preview/mmwrhtml/rr5514a1.htm.

Brown, W. J., and A. Singhal. 1999. "Entertainment-Education Strategies for Social Change." In *Mass Media, Social Control and Social Change.* D. P. Demers and K. Viswanath, eds. Ames, Iowa: Iowa State University Press: 263–280.

Brown, William J., Benson P. Fraser, and Steven Kiruswa. 2004. "Promoting HIV/AIDS Prevention through Dramatic Film: Lessons from Tanzania and Kenya." Paper presented to the Fourth International Conference on Entertainment-Education for Social Change. Durban, South Africa, September 26–30.

Centers for Disease Control and Prevention (CDC). 2003. "Advancing HIV Prevention: New Strategies for a Changing Epidemic—United States, 2003." *Morbidity and Mortality Weekly Report (MMWR).* April 18. 52, 15:329–332. CDC Web site. Accessed online December 2008. http://www.cdc.gov/mmwr/preview/mmwrhtml/mm5215a1.htm.

———. 2006. "Evolution of HIV/AIDS Prevention Programs—United States, 1981–2006." *Morbidity and Mortality Weekly Report (MMWR).* June 2. 55, 21:597–603. CDC Web site. Accessed online December 2008. http://www.cdc.gov/mmwR/preview/mmwrhtml/mm5521a4.htm.

———. 2007. "Rapid HIV Testing in Outreach and Other Community Settings—United States, 2004–2006." *Morbidity and Mortality Weekly Report (MMWR).* November 30. 56, 47:1233–1237. CDC Web site. Accessed online December 2008. http://www.cdc.gov/mmwr/preview/mmwrhtml/mm5647a2.htm?s_cid=mm5647a2_e.

———. 2008a. "HIV Testing." CDC Web Site. Accessed online December 2008. http://www.cdc.gov/hiv/topics/testing/.

———. 2008b. "Persons Tested for HIV—United States, 2006." *Morbidity and Mortality Weekly Report (MMWR).* August 8. 57, 31:845–849. CDC Web site. Accessed online December 2008. http://www.cdc.gov/mmwr/preview/mmwrhtml/mm5731a1.htm.

DiClemente, Ralph J., and Richard A. Crosby. 2006. "Preventing HIV Infection in Adolescents: What Works for Uninfected Teens." In *Teenagers, HIV, and AIDS: Insights from Youths Living with the Virus.* Lyon, Maureen E., and Lawrence J. D'Angelo, eds. Westport, CT: Praeger:143–161.

"The Digital Opportunity: Using New Media for Public Education Campaigns." 2007. Forum hosted by the Ad Council and the Kaiser Family Foundation. July 19. The Kaiser Family Foundation Web site. Accessed online November 2008. http://www.kff.org/entmedia/entmedia071907pkg.cfm.

Food and Drug Administration (FDA)/Center for Biologics Evaluation and Research. "Testing Yourself for HIV-1, the Virus that Causes AIDS." FDA Web site. Accessed online December 2008. http://www.fda.gov/CbER/infosheets/hiv-home2.htm.

Global HIV Prevention Working Group. 2007. "Bringing HIV Prevention to Scale: An Urgent Global Priority." Global HIV Prevention Working Group. Kaiser Family Foundation Web Site. Accessed online December 2008. http://www.kff.org/hivaids/ hiv062807pkg.cfm.

Greenwald, Jeffrey L., Gale R. Burstein, Jonathan Pincus, and Bernard Branson. 2006. "A Rapid Review of Rapid HIV Antibody Tests." *Current Infectious Disease Reports.* 8:125–131. CDC Web site. Accessed online December 2008. http://www.cdc.gov/hiv/ topics/testing/resources/journal_article/pdf/rapid_review.pdf.

Health Communication Partnership. 2006. "South African HIV/AIDS Serial Drama Helps Decrease Stigma and Improve Prevention Behaviors Among Youth." *Communication Impact!* Johns Hopkins University, Center for Communication Programs. Accessed online September 2008. http://www.jhuccp.org/pubs/ci/20/20.pdf.

Holtgrave, D., and T. Anderson. 2004. "Utilizing HIV Transmission Rates to Assist in Prioritizing HIV Prevention Services." International Journal of STDs and AIDS. 15, 12:789–792.

Kaiser Family Foundation. 2000. National Survey of Teens on HIV/AIDS 2000. Menlo Park, CA: Kaiser Family Foundation. Accessed online September 2008. http://www. kff.org/youthhivstds/upload/National-Survey-of-Teens-on-HIV-AIDS.pdf.

School Health Policies and Programs Study (SHPPS). 2007. *Journal of School Health.* 77, 8. October 2007 edition of journal devoted to comprehensive discussion of SHPPS.

Sexuality Information and Education Council of the United States (SIECUS). 2007. "SIECUS Public Policy Office Fact Sheet: What the Research Says." October. SIECUS Web site. Accessed December 2008. http://www.siecus.org/_data/global/images/ research_says.pdf.

Shapiro, D., D. Meekers, and B. Tambashe. 2003. "Exposure to the '*SIDA dans la Cité*' AIDS Prevention Television Series in Côte d'Ivoire, Sexual Risk Behaviour and Condom Use." *AIDS Care.* 15, 3:303–314.

Sternberg, Steve. 2006. "AIDS Drives Plots on TV." *USA Today.* August 7. Accessed online September 2008. http://www.usatoday.com/life/television/news/2006-08-07-aids-on-tv_x.htm.

Underhill, Kristen, Paul Montgomery, and Don Operario. 2007. "Sexual Abstinence Only Programmes to Prevent HIV Infection in High Income Countries: Systematic Review." *BMJ (British Medical Journal).* 335, 7613:248–259.

PART II

Issues Surrounding HIV/AIDS

CHAPTER 5

Social Perceptions
of HIV/AIDS

In this chapter, we will look at

- How HIV/AIDS has been impacted by stigmatized views of the virus and of those who are infected
- Factors shaping social perceptions of HIV/AIDS
- Public opinion data on HIV/AIDS

WHAT ARE THE SOCIAL PERCEPTIONS OF HIV/AIDS AND THOSE WHO ARE HIV+?

Various factors other than physical symptoms and objective signs of illness (like a fever or a rash) color the way we think about a particular disease and those who have it. Patient characteristics (such as race, age, sex, and social class) and the epidemiology of the disease (patterns of where and how the disease spreads) are just as important as the diagnosis, prognosis, cause, and treatment. Also, those who play some role of dealing with the disease or communicating about it to others (like physicians or patient advocacy groups) play a role in how a disease is perceived and how people react to those who have it (Duffin, 2005). All of these factors come into play in forming social perceptions about HIV/AIDS and those who are HIV+.

The Social Construction of HIV/AIDS

To fully understand HIV and AIDS, it necessary to look at how the virus and people who are infected with it have been perceived by others in

society. This means we need to understand that AIDS is a socially constructed illness. The term "social construction" means that as people interact (social) with each other, they create or build (construct) an
understanding of reality (how the world is). They create and accept ideas
about situations or categories of people. Their actions then begin to support that perspective. From the beginning of the pandemic, HIV/AIDS has
been socially constructed in stigmatizing ways resulting in negative perceptions of the virus and those who have it, as well as resulting in behaviors that reflect that stigmatization.

HIV/AIDS-related stigma is "a term that refers to prejudice, discount-
ing, discrediting, and discrimination directed at people perceived to have
AIDS or HIV, and the individuals, groups, and communities with which
they are associated" (Herek, 1999, 1106). Such stigmas have been documented in varying forms throughout the world, ranging from personal
attacks to loss of jobs or homes to discriminatory legislation. These stigmas even impact the behavior of people who have HIV/AIDS themselves
and those associated with them.

Sociologist Peter Conrad (1990) argues that the way Americans view
and respond to HIV/AIDS has been shaped by a social construction that
actually built a triple stigma. First, from the beginning, HIV/AIDS was
connected with socially stigmatized groups. Second, HIV is sexually
transmitted. Third, until advances in treatment well into the second decade
of the pandemic, AIDS was a terminal, wasting disease. Each of these
stigmas can be examined in turn.

Socially stigmatized groups. First, the early emphasis by most American
epidemiologists, physicians, and researchers focused on AIDS as a disease
of male homosexuals and intravenous drug users. The result was that they
constructed AIDS in such a way that the disease, and thereby those
infected with HIV, became associated with marginalized behaviors. If they
had looked through a broader lens on the growing pandemic, they would
have not limited their focus so narrowly. They would have acknowledged
the known cases of women and infants with AIDS, for example, and the
largely heterosexual nature of AIDS transmission in Africa and elsewhere
(Wright, 2006).

Following their lead, the association of HIV/AIDS with homosexuality
and drugs proliferated among those outside of the medical arena. For
example, partially through selective reporting, the mass media perpetu-
ated this stigma (e.g., Altman, 1986; Albert, 1986; Baker, 1986; Cook and
Colby, 1992; Kinsella, 1989). Conservative religious leaders publicly pro-
claimed AIDS to be God's judgment on homosexuals and on society (e.g.,

Engel, 2006:69–75). In the federal government, the conservative political administration of Ronald Reagan (U.S. President, 1981–1989) was also accused of being slow to respond to the growing AIDS crisis because of this association with homosexuality and drug use (e.g., Shilts, 1987). Reagan himself did not even publicly use the word "AIDS" until 1985, four years after the CDC's first report in the summer of 1981 (see the primary source document "President Ronald Reagan's First Public Statement on AIDS" in Appendix B). AIDS Activist Larry Kramer (1987) went so far as to call the Reagan administration's reaction "genocide" against homosexuals. The impact of HIV/AIDS and the way it was being shaped by these and other powerful entities reverberated across society.

Another perhaps less obvious aspect of this "social construction" of a disease involves its name:

> A disease concept blends ideas about the illness and ideas about the people who are likely to suffer from it . . . A name or diagnosis is crucial. It provides a label, an identity, an organizing principle for further discussion. Usually a disease concept is born with its first name, although the associated illness may have been recognized long before. Having been named, a disease takes on a distinct life of its own, separate from other diseases (Duffin, 2005: 8, 11).

Not only does the name of a disease impact our thinking, but also our familiarity with the disease or with those who currently have it shapes our views. Such connections also determine whether our thoughts about the disease are detached or more emotional (Duffin, 2005). The initial association of HIV/AIDS with male homosexuality was emphasized through the early names for the disease that predate AIDS such as "Gay-Related Immunodeficiency" (commonly referred to by the acronym GRID), the "gay cancer," and the "gay plague." Another early name, the "4-H Disease," also incorporated additional stigmatized groups identified with the disease: homosexuals, heroin users, Haitian immigrants, and hemophiliacs. Sometimes "hookers" were included rather than hemophiliacs. Stigma and discrimination that remain against HIV/AIDS and those who have HIV/AIDS still often refers back to these early constructions.

Sexual transmission. Most diseases are categorized and named by their characteristics or effects. Sexually transmitted infections (STIs), however, are categorized by how they are transmitted. HIV can be transmitted through sexual activity but not through casual contact (see Chapter 1). Sexually transmitted infections, and those who have them, have long been the subject of negative moral judgments and stigmas. The turn of the

twentieth century, for example, saw a "general hysteria" about STIs. Doctors even differentiated between "innocent" victims of STIs (*venereal
insontium*), such as newborns blinded from gonorrhea, and others (Brandt,
1988: 148).

The sexual component of HIV/AIDS is compounded in that stigma is
also more likely to occur when a disease is perceived as the responsibility
of the person who has it. HIV/AIDS is largely transmitted through behaviors that are seen as voluntary as well as promiscuous, immoral, or deviant
(Herek, 1999). As Harvard historian Allan Brandt observed of the
early years of the AIDS epidemic:

> Social values continue to define sexually transmitted diseases as uniquely
> sinful and, indeed, to transform them into evidence of moral decay; some
> still believe that fear of disease encourages a higher morality . . . underlying
> tensions in American sexual values persist, tensions that are brought for-
> ward in our approach to AIDS as well as to venereal diseases. To conserva-
> tive foes of the sexual revolution, the message is clear: The way to control
> sexually transmitted disease is not through medical means but through
> moral rectitude. A disease such as AIDS is controlled by controlling
> individual conduct (1988: 166).

In the late 1980s, stigma interrupted scientifically sound attempts to
research sexual behaviors among American adults and teenagers that may
have helped better understand and address the growing HIV/AIDS epidemic in the United States. Two studies were planned, the Survey of Health
and AIDS Risk Prevalence (SHARP) and the American Teenage Study
(ATS). Both were designed and approved by some of the preeminent social
scientists in the country and funded by the prestigious National Institutes
of Health for almost $20 million each. However, conservative politicians
intervened and the research was ultimately blocked (Udry, 1993).

Research on the medical and social aspects of HIV/AIDS has taken
huge strides forward since those studies were interrupted; however, there
are still huge gaps in knowledge. Two decades later, for example,
researchers would continue to assess that "little empirical data exist within
the United States to characterize men who purchase sex or to assess their
sexual risk and HIV/STI infection" (Decker et al., 2008). Although attitudes toward HIV/AIDS are changing as discussed below, stigmas surrounding the perception of sexually transmitted infections, including
HIV/AIDS, still work in shaping the pandemic worldwide.

Disease characteristics. Throughout history, epidemic and deadly diseases
have caused incredible fear. This fear has been especially acute when the
cause of the disease, routes of transmission, danger of contagion, or cure

have been unknown. Lethality also plays a role in assigning stigma, because those diseases considered fatal receive the greatest stigma. Additionally, conditions that are disfiguring, obvious, or uncomfortably perceived by others are more highly stigmatized (Herek, 1999). Fears and discrimination often focus on those who are ill and those accused of spreading disease. Leprosy, for example, fit each of these criteria, evoking fear, stigma, and ostracism of the afflicted throughout history.

From the earliest days through most of the second decade of the pandemic, AIDS was considered fatal. In its final stages, AIDS is also a wasting disease. The victims lose a great amount of weight and suffer from a variety of opportunistic illnesses such as the distinctive skin lesions of Kaposi's Sarcoma that make their deteriorating physical condition obvious. Only in the late 1990s did advances in antiretroviral medication begin somewhat to quell fear about certain fatality by extending the life spans and quality of life for many living with HIV infection or who had been diagnosed with AIDS. However, medications are not a magic bullet against the virus. Especially in countries where medications are not widely available, the perception—and reality—of the severity of HIV/AIDS remains.

PUBLIC OPINION ON HIV/AIDS

What do public opinion polls reveal about views of HIV/AIDS and those who are infected? In 2006, 42% of Americans reported that they personally know someone who has or had died from AIDS or is HIV+ (Kaiser Family Foundation, 2008c). Forty-five percent of Americans agreed that there is "a lot of discrimination" in the United States against people with HIV and AIDS. This percentage has varied only slightly since the mid-1980s (Kaiser Family Foundation, 2008a). Fifty percent of respondents also said that the HIV/AIDS epidemic has made people more likely to discriminate against gays and lesbians (Kaiser Family Foundation, 2008a). Respondents were also asked, "When you think about HIV/AIDS, which group of people do you think of first as those who are most likely to be infected?" The question was "open-ended," meaning that no answers were provided for the choices; respondents could list whichever groups came to mind. Forty-three percent identified gay males as their response, indicating that the social construction of HIV/AIDS as largely impacting gays still colors public perceptions of the epidemic in the United States (Kaiser Family Foundation, 2008c).

Stigma also appeared to be related to respondents' knowledge about HIV/AIDS. For example, 76% of those who knew correctly that HIV cannot be transmitted through a drinking glass reported that they would be very or somewhat comfortable working with a person who has HIV; only 53% of those who incorrectly believed that HIV could be transmitted through a drinking glass agreed. A similar percentage (77%) who correctly knew that HIV cannot be transmitted by touching a toilet seat also agreed with the statement, compared to only 42% of those who thought HIV could be transmitted in that manner (Kaiser Family Foundation, 2008a).

Overall, however, public opinion data reveal a somewhat more complicated picture of the HIV/AIDS pandemic. Overall concern about HIV/AIDS among Americans has shown a dramatic decline since the mid-1990s. In 1995, 44% of Americans identified HIV/AIDS as the most urgent health problem facing the nation. That percentage had dropped significantly to only 17% by 2002, where it remained (after some minor fluctuation) in 2006 (Kaiser Family Foundation, 2008c). In contrast, between 2000 and 2006, roughly one-third of Americans polled continued to rate HIV/AIDs as the most urgent health problem globally (Kaiser Family Foundation, 2008b).

Likely reflecting the demographic realities of the populations most impacted by HIV/AIDS, concern varies by race, ethnicity, and age. African Americans and Latinos, two groups that have seen a troublesome rise in incidence of HIV/AIDS over this time period, were far more likely than whites to rank HIV/AIDS as the nation's most urgent health problem (39% for African Americans; 23% for Latinos; only 13% for whites). African Americans and Latinos were also somewhat more likely than whites to identify HIV/AIDS as the most urgent global health problem (44%, 43%, and 30% respectively). A notable decline (from 55% in 1995 to 34% in 2006) among African Americans expressing personal concerns about becoming infected with HIV has occurred; however, African Americans and Latinos (at 31%) remained more concerned than whites (at 9%) on this matter (Kaiser Family Foundation, 2008c).

Similarly, younger adults were far more likely than older adults to list HIV/AIDS as the most urgent health problem facing the United States. Twenty-eight percent of those aged 18–29 listed HIV/AIDS compared to only 10% of those in the 65+ age range (Kaiser Family Foundation, 2008c). This finding reflects not only long-standing albeit increasingly misplaced perceptions that HIV/AIDS is primarily a concern only for young adults, but the reality that half of all new HIV infections occur among this age group.

Americans overall were more likely in 2006 than in 1995 to say that the United States is making progress in the HIV/AIDS epidemic (40%

compared to 32% respectively) (Kaiser Family Foundation, 2008c). They were divided as to whether the same trend holds globally. Forty percent indicated they think the world is "losing ground" while 36% said the world is "making progress" (Kaiser Family Foundation, 2008b).

Americans were also generally in support of spending federal monies to combat HIV/AIDS in 2006, with 63% agreeing that "too little" is spent on HIV/AIDS in the United States. That is up from 51% who agreed with that position in 1995. Across the same period of time, those saying that the United States spends "too much" on the domestic problem of HIV/AIDS (only 7% in 2006) has remained relatively stable (Kaiser Family Foundation, 2008c). The majority of respondents also generally agreed that domestic federal spending on HIV/AIDS prevention and testing would lead to progress (62% and 59% respectively) (Kaiser Family Foundation, 2008c).

Looking globally, 56% of respondents agreed that the United States is spending "too little" to deal with HIV/AIDS in developing countries, and the majority (60%) felt that such spending would lead to meaningful progress (Kaiser Family Foundation, 2008b). Yet, other groups were also identified as "not doing enough" to fight HIV/AIDS in the developing world, including governments in countries hardest hit by the pandemic (76%), pharmaceutical companies (64%), governments of other developed nations (54%), and international nonprofit organizations and foundations (46%) (Kaiser Family Foundation, 2008b).

Overall, a lack of funds from the United States and other developed nations was cited by fewer people (43%) as a reason why it has been difficult to control the spread of HIV/AIDS in developing countries than those who cited reasons of widespread poverty (78%), corruption or misuse of funding (71%), lack of efforts from those nations' governments (75%) and the "unwillingness of people in developing countries to change their unsafe sexual practices" (74%). The last item is notable in that it is the only one that places blame for the ongoing pandemic at the individual behavioral level. It is also notable because, when forced to choose among these reasons to select only one as most important, almost one-third of all respondents (30%) chose this item. That was a larger percentage than chose any other response, even widespread poverty, which garnered 23% agreement as the second most chosen reason (Kaiser Family Foundation, 2008b).

REFERENCES

Albert, Edward. 1986. "Illness and Deviance: The Response of the Press to AIDS." In *The Social Dimensions of AIDS: Method and Theory*. Douglas A. Feldman and Thomas M. Johnson, eds. New York: Praeger, 163–178.

Altman, Dennis. 1986. *AIDS in the Mind of America*. New York: Anchor.

Baker, Andrea J. 1986. "The Portrayal of AIDS in the Media: An Analysis of Articles in the *New York Times*." In *The Social Dimensions of AIDS: Method and Theory*. Douglas A. Feldman and Thomas M. Johnson, eds. New York: Praeger, 179–194.

Brandt, Allan M. 1988. "AIDS: From Social History to Social Policy." In *AIDS: The Burdens of History*. Elizabeth Fee and Daniel M. Fox, editors. Berkeley: University of California Press, 147–168. Accessed online October 2008. http://ark.cdlib.org/ark:/13030/ft7t1nb59n/.

Conrad, Peter. 1990. "The Social Stigma of AIDS." In *Sociology of Health and Illness: Critical Perspectives*, 3rd edition. Peter Conrad and Rochelle Kern, eds. New York: St. Martin's Press, 285–292.

Cook, Timothy E., and David C. Colby. 1992. "The Mass-Mediated Epidemic: The Politics of AIDS on the Nightly Network News." *AIDS: The Making of a Chronic Disease*. Elizabeth Fee and Daniel M. Fox, eds. Berkeley: University of Chicago Press: 84–122.

Decker, M.R., A. Raj, J. Gupta, and J.G. Silverman. 2008. "Sex Purchasing and Associations with HIV/STI Among a Clinic-Based Sample of U.S. Men." *Journal of Acquired Immune Deficiency Syndromes (JAIDS)*. 48, 3: 355–59.

Doka, Kenneth J. 1997. *AIDS, Fear, and Society: Challenging the Dreaded Disease*. Bristol, PA: Taylor & Francis.

Duffin, Jacalyn. 2005. *Lovers and Livers: Disease Concepts in History*. Toronto: University of Toronto Press.

Engel, Jonathan. 2006. *The Epidemic: A Global History of AIDS*. New York: Smithsonian Books/Collins.

Herek, Gregory. 1999. "AIDS and Stigma." *American Behavioral Scientist*. 42, 7:1106–16.

Kaiser Family Foundation. 2008a. "Attitudes About Stigma and Discrimination Related to HIV/AIDS." Accessed online November 2008. http://www.kff.org/spotlight/hivstigma/index.cfm.

_____. 2008b. "Public Opinion on the Global HIV/AIDS Epidemic." Accessed online November 2008. http://www.kff.org/spotlight/hivglobal/index.cfm.

_____. 2008c. "Public Opinion on the HIV/AIDS Epidemic in the United States." Accessed online November 2008. http://www.kff.org/spotlight/hivUS/index.cfm

Kinsella, James. 1989. *Covering the Plague: AIDS and the American Media*. New Brunswick, NJ: Rutgers University Press.

Kramer, Larry. 1991. (orig. 1987). "The Plague Years." *The AIDS Reader: Social, Ethical, Political Issues*. Nancy F. McKenzie, ed. New York: Meridian.

Shilts, Randy. 1987. *And the Band Played On: Politics, People, and the AIDS Epidemic*. New York: St. Martin's Press.

Udry, J.R. 1993. "The Politics of Sex Research." *The Journal of Sex Research*. 30:103–110.

Wright, Eric R. 2006. "The Social Construction of AIDS." In *Teaching the Sociology of HIV/AIDS*, 3rd ed. Carrie E. Foote-Ardah and Eric R. Wright, compilers and editors. New York: American Sociological Association, 194–213.

CHAPTER 6

Social Action on HIV/AIDS

In this chapter, we will

- Introduce a model of social action
- Use that model to better understand collective social responses to HIV/AIDS
- Discuss the difficulty of initiating massive social change

When a virulent pandemic like HIV/AIDS emerges in a society or globally, drastic social action is needed to reduce the impact. Unlike other viruses or diseases, there is no vaccination or cure for HIV/AIDS, so a "simple" solution of inoculations could not be administered on such a massive scale. When these limitations are recognized, the task of reducing the spread and impact of a pandemic like HIV/AIDS becomes much more challenging. The monumental task then becomes getting millions of people to change their everyday behavior. This is not easy to do.

One of the best models for understanding how this process works has been developed by sociologist Joel Best (Best, 2008). Best has identified a six-step process that occurs within industrialized societies that transforms a seemingly minor social issue into a significant social problem. We will use Best's six-step process to identify what has occurred with social responses to HIV/AIDS within the last twenty five years or so.

THE SIX-STAGE PROCESS

Best (2008) argues that there are six stages to what he calls the "Basic Natural History Model of the Social Problems Process." The stages, even though they appear in linear order, do not necessarily have to unfold that way. In other words, even though analytically it appears that there is a

linear progression from one stage to the next, each stage is not a necessary
and sufficient condition for the emergence of the next stage nor any of the
future stages. Generally, however each stage does occur and generally
occurs in this order:

1. Claimsmaking
2. Media Coverage
3. Public Reaction
4. Policymaking
5. Social Problems Work
6. Policy Outcomes

We will review the characteristics of each stage briefly and discuss the
characteristics of each stage in the course of the HIV/AIDS pandemic
becoming recognized as a serious social and global problem.

Claimsmaking

Claimsmaking is precisely what it appears to be; the making of claims
about a particular condition that needs to be recognized as a social problem. Claims can be made by experts and activists. In either case, the claim
is essentially an argument that calls attention to a troubling condition and
attempts to make the case that "this is a serious problem." In regards to
HIV/AIDS, the argument for both being problems has tragically become
easier as the numbers of people infected with HIV, living with HIV/AIDS
and dying due to AIDS has grown considerably, along with the general
public's awareness of these numbers. In a very sad way, the case for
HIV/AIDS being recognized as a serious social problem occurred without
much need for specific claimsmaking.

The exceptions to this were the claims made about the seriousness of
HIV/AIDS when it was still considered to be a "gay" problem. Recall that
when first identified by the CDC in 1981, the initial AIDS cases consisted
of five gay men; as such, there was no immediate concern to take large-
scale social action, in part because researchers and physicians were initially unclear as to what the cause was.

After HIV was identified as the causal factor in the development of
AIDS, essentially, two claims began to be made. First, that even though
HIV/AIDS seemed to be primarily confined to the gay, male population,
those members still deserved the same amount of due consideration and
treatment response as any other group. This claim was generally made by
gay activists and others concerned with social justice. The second claim,
generally made by those in the health field, was that even though
HIV/AIDS may have initially been confined to the gay male population,

there was considerable potential for it to spread to the heterosexual population. This claim originated once the methods of transmission were identified. The first claim is significant historically as there was a fair amount of public discourse on HIV/AIDS with religious overtones; for example, this was retribution from God, it was a way that God was going to rid the world of gays, and so forth. The second claim was equally as relevant, because it is well known that many people are neither exclusively gay nor exclusively straight—their sexual partners come from both groups; as such there was an acknowledgment that a high likelihood existed for HIV/AIDS to spread beyond just the gay community. In addition, there was the threat of HIV transmission from both sex workers and intravenous drug users (IDUs).

Once the potential for transmission was fully appreciated, the numbers of people (both hetero- and homosexual) testing positive for HIV began to increase, and the knowledge that there was very little effective treatment and that neither HIV nor AIDS had a cure was disseminated, the recognition of the pandemic being a serious social problem was easily understood.

Media Coverage

The second stage in this process is the extent to which the media covers the claim. The more coverage that it receives, the greater the chance that it will be considered serious by more people. Recall that the original intent of this "social-probleming" process is collective social action toward some goal. In the case of HIV/AIDS, the goal is getting people to change their behavior, whether that behavior is IDU, unprotected sex, not getting tested, and so on. The overall outcome of this type of social action is to get people to stop or reduce negative or dangerous behaviors and increase positive, healthy behaviors. Before people can even consider changing their behavior, however, they need to recognize that they are engaging in a problematic behavior. Generally this is achieved through public education efforts that utilize the power of various media. Briefly, if media outlets are reporting on it (both national and local), then it must be a problem. "If it is a problem and it is something that I am doing, then I must be engaging in problematic behavior. I should consider changing it." Developing such an attitude would be the expected outcome of media coverage.

As the seriousness of the HIV/AIDS pandemic grew, the government and other concerned organizations began to develop public awareness campaigns specifically designed to reduce the risk of HIV transmission and prevent AIDS. These included news stories on HIV/AIDS, documentaries, movies, pamphlets, public service announcements (with and without celebrities), HIV/AIDS awareness education in schools and other public settings, adding universal precaution trainings on HIV transmission for health care workers, and inclusion of HIV/AIDS educational programming in substance abuse treatment settings among others. These efforts at using the media to forward critical, life-saving information have proven to be successful, as more people are far more aware of HIV/AIDS, risk of infection, routes of transmission, and other related issues than at any time in the past. This is not to say that they need to stop, however; each new generation of individuals needs to be exposed to the same information so as to continue to lower the risk of HIV infection.

Public Reaction

Effective claimsmaking and media coverage result in concern among the general public for the emerging social problem. Public reaction is crucial in determining the success of the social action (see chapters 5 and 7). If the public is concerned about the issue, then there is a good chance that problematic behavior on a collective level can change. Effective media coverage results in people talking about the issue more often with more people. Prior to a media campaign some members of the public may have been completely unaware of the issue. Once various media facilitate information about the issue, it enters into daily public discourse, and more and more people begin to talk about it with family members and friends, thus spreading knowledge about the issue and establishing it as a social concern. The media bring the issue forward through various channels and then members of the public, influenced by the fact that the issue is deserving of media attention, begin to talk about it, disseminating it and saturating it as a topic of discussion within daily discourse.

As noted, HIV/AIDS was originally not thought to be a threat to anyone who wasn't gay, or more specifically, anyone who wasn't male and gay. As such, there was little concern for heterosexual males or females about contracting the virus. In addition, information on the routes of transmission was limited, and many people who thought they were members of a low-risk population did not take any precautions. Once more was known about HIV and its transmission and this information was disseminated through the efforts of the media, public reaction changed from one of mild concern to troubling concern. Many recognized that even though they were not identified as belonging to a high-risk group, virtually anyone was capable of becoming HIV positive. Put simply, once the threat of HIV/AIDS went from seemingly low risk to high risk, it became personal for many people; once people have a personal stake in a social issue, the collective level of concern for social action increases.

Policymaking

It is well acknowledged that one of the best ways to change the behavior of large numbers of people is through the establishment of policies. In highly industrialized and rational societies, people are trained early on to attend and respond to policies implemented by various institutions. In other words, by creating policies, governmental and other organizational bodies can regulate the behavior of collectivities of people. By establishing policies, they can also clarify what is considered to be problematic; if a policy about something has been enacted, it is generally because whatever that something is has been problematic in the past and remains so currently. (Chapter 7 covers some specific policies addressing HIV/AIDS.)

One of the bodies that exercises great control over large numbers of people is the government—more specifically the regulatory agencies at all levels of organization (federal to local). Since all people are socialized to respond to governmental directives and initiatives, many people easily respond to policies regulating behavior that are established by the government. The manifest purpose of governmental policies is to ameliorate the social issue that required the policy in the first place. As such, governments around the world in conjunction with the medical community have developed and implemented policies about many aspects relating to HIV/AIDS.

There is insufficient space to discuss all of the policies implemented in response to HIV/AIDS. Suffice it say that those that have been enacted have attempted to respond to the prevention, intervention and treatment of HIV/AIDS. The extent to which they have been effective is in part based on the extent to which people have behaved in accordance with them; this hearkens back to the need for various media to make the policies and their respective implications known to the general public. Overall, however, most efforts at policymaking in relation to HIV/AIDS have been effective.

Social Problems Work

Once policies have been established, implementation of their nuts and bolts follows. This is where the ideal policy outcome and the real challenge of changing behavior on a large scale meet; in most cases, the reality of the implementation of the policy is much different than the anticipated outcome. This is not to say that it is not possible to achieve desired outcomes, nor is it to criticize efforts by social change workers to effect positive change; rather it is an acknowledgment that social-change

---

HIV/AIDS ADVOCACY

Below is a brief list of organizations that advocate for many issues related to HIV/AIDS.

ACT UP
http://www.actupny.org

AIDS Action
http://www.aidsaction.org

Project Inform
http://www.projectinform.org

The Body
http://www.thebody.com/index.html

World AIDS Day
http://www.worldaidscampaign.org

---

work is difficult and demanding, and many times the final outcomes of a policy are not those that were planned.

This work is also challenging due to system dynamics. This means that the way that society is organized is like a system of parts that work together to maintain the whole. A current buzzword for this dynamic is "interconnected." Change in one area or component of a system inevitably brings change in other parts of the system, the entire system, or both. The problem lies in any individual or collectivity's ability to predict what those changes might be and how they might affect the overall system, the other components of the system, or even the component that has been changed. So it is entirely possible that some social change work can result in an even greater social problem than the one that was targeted for change.

In regards to HIV/AIDS, we can observe the social problems and social change work in the forms of public education, more funding opportunities for research on prevention, intervention and treatment, federal protections of medical records of anyone HIV positive, syringe-exchange programs, increased funding for AIDS medications throughout the world, international participation in reducing HIV/AIDS throughout the world, and so forth. All of these efforts have resulted from the recognition of HIV/AIDS as a global pandemic that requires coordinated governmental intervention, institutional policymaking, and comprehensive social change efforts.

One can gain an appreciation of the impact that HIV/AIDS has had (and continues to have) globally when one considers the fact that despite all of these efforts, despite the billions of dollars spent, despite the thousands of hours of education, despite the hundreds of thousands of lives lost due to HIV/AIDS, it still remains a problem. Note that the problem is partly due to our current inability to vaccinate against HIV and to "cure" AIDS, but the bulk of the problem has been and remains, getting millions of people to engage in different behaviors. Behavioral change is crucial as a response to HIV/AIDS because it is clearly established that it is behavior that transmits the virus. Unfortunately, massive behavior change is a very difficult outcome to achieve.

Policy Outcomes

As noted above, not all policy outcomes are those that were anticipated. And as with all government initiatives and all institutional efforts at broad-based social change, not all people will be convinced that the policy or the change was sufficient, comprehensive enough, or equitable for all parties. One factor that contributes to the efficacy of any attempts at large-scale social change is the availability of resources to effect the change. Inevitably necessary resources are lacking or limited. As such, efforts at policy implementation and social change cannot always be as thorough as intended. Similarly, as also noted above, change in one component of the system can result in unexpected changes in other components, thus sometimes aggravating the original problem and, in turn, creating more problems that require attention.

What is required for a reasonable determination of the efficacy of any social change effort or policy outcome is ongoing monitoring and evaluation of the initiative. Most sources funding social change efforts today require an evaluation component to determine if the anticipated changes are occurring and if not, determine how the effort can adapt or be modified to result in those changes. These efforts require resources as well, and again, in many cases, the resources available are insufficient or lacking, and effective evaluation methods are compromised.

The above discussion applies to all aspects of HIV/AIDS work conducted. Some have argued that the governmental response to HIV/AIDS was too slow, policies were ineffective, organizational support was initially too limited. It is difficult to determine the accuracy of many of these claims, because historical decision-making always needs to be made in context. When it comes to governmental decision-making, knowing the full context of what went into any decisions made about HIV/AIDS is very difficult. It is clear, however, that much more could have been done

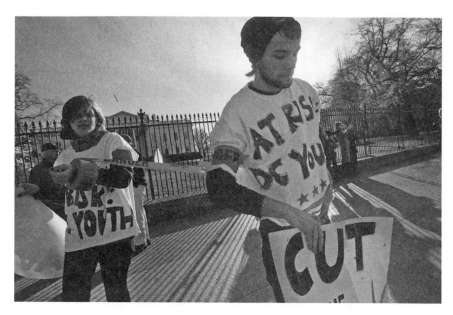

Figure 6.1 Students from the George Washington University chapter of the Student Global AIDS Campaign wrap themselves in red tape during a 2007 protest outside the White House, calling on the federal government to "cut the red tape" around access to AIDS prevention and treatment. (AP Photo/Jacquelyn Martin.)

early on, when HIV/AIDS had limited impact. Of course, this too is a controversial claim to make in and of itself as the full range of scientific knowledge about HIV/AIDS was limited. In any event, there is much greater knowledge of the relative effectiveness of various strategies in the prevention, intervention, and treatment of HIV/AIDS. Because the knowledge base is greater, efforts to determine policy outcomes are more substantial.

With some measures (efficacy of antiretroviral medication) outcomes are easier to measure than others (efficacy of public education encouraging condom use, reduction in the sharing of syringes, increased testing for HIV, and the like), however. This is due to the ability to collect data on certain outcomes with higher levels of accuracy and control than on others. Collecting data on viral load for large numbers of HIV-positive persons for example, is fairly easy, because those data are collected in the normal course of treatment and in fact, are used to determine efficacy of current treatment regimens. Collecting data on the number of people that are using substances intravenously and sharing syringes, however, is far more difficult to obtain due to the fact this is an ongoing behavior and is not readily amenable to observation. In order to determine how many people are IDU's and how often they share syringes with others would require constant surveillance of an entire population of people; it is unlikely that this would ever happen. Generally, most policy outcomes are determined from data that are collected indirectly; many are simply claims by experts, government representatives, or others about the efficacy of the policy.

SUMMARY

Large-scale social action is very difficult to conduct for most groups and organizations due to the limitation of resources. A global pandemic like HIV/AIDS, however, can motivate large numbers of people to engage in social action due to its tragic and irreversible consequences; in this case, the resources were and continue to be forthcoming. The question as to how effective any social action is in successfully changing social behavior on a massive scale is difficult to determine with precision. It is easy to say, however, that the resources expended to reduce the spread of HIV and ameliorate the impact of AIDS have saved many people much suffering. HIV and AIDS are fairly well entrenched in the vocabularies of most people due to the social action work that has been conducted, this too is quite an achievement and in and of itself, is reflective of effective social change work.

REFERENCE

Best, Joel. 2008. *Social Problems*. New York: W.W. Norton.

CHAPTER 7

Policy Responses to HIV/AIDS

In this chapter, we will look at

- The impact of stigma and discrimination on those with HIV/AIDS and those close to them
- Federal policy protections against HIV/AIDS-related discrimination
- Federal policies providing other forms of support for the HIV/AIDS community

Various policies have been enacted to respond to the needs of those with HIV/AIDS and their families. Many of these policy responses are at the state level and vary from state to state. Here, we discuss a selection of federal policy responses to HIV/AIDS.

THE IMPACT OF HIV/AIDS-RELATED STIGMA AND DISCRIMINATION

One of the difficult social problems people with HIV/AIDS have to deal with is the negative stigma long associated with the disease. (Chapter 5 discusses this issue in more detail.) The impact of stigma on those with HIV/AIDS or somehow connected to HIV/AIDS can have severe consequences for individuals with HIV. When stigma results from assigning "guilt" (e.g., drug users or prostitutes) versus "innocence" (e.g., an HIV+ infant), discrimination against those judged "guilty" may be especially acute (Pollak, Paicheler, and Pierret, 1992: 18–22).

Stigma can even impact the behaviors of those who have or suspect they have HIV/AIDS themselves. A study by Anish P. Mahajan and coauthors (2008) supported previous research in affirming that, even well into the third decade of the AIDS pandemic, stigma has still discouraged or deterred people from being tested for HIV; disclosing their HIV status to sexual partners and others; seeking information, health care and medications; and maintaining medication regimens. Additionally, efforts aimed at prevention, education, and testing must address stigma to be effective; unfortunately, many such programs do not do so.

AIDS SERVICE ORGANIZATIONS

When individuals learn that they are infected with HIV, they have enormous emotions to face, decisions to make, health information to learn, and potentially large related financial costs to bear. They may need social supports in each of these areas. AIDS service organizations (ASOs) can be valuable resources, especially for the newly diagnosed. These organizations "help people connect with the information and resources they need" (ASO Spotlight, 2007: 22) including resources as diverse as health care and medications, food, housing, counseling, support groups, addiction treatments, transportation, financial planning needs, and even legal representation. They are staffed by experts who know what benefits, resources, and options are available and how to access what people with HIV need. ASOs are often listed in the yellow pages of telephone directories under "AIDS" or "Social Service Organizations" or can be found through online searches (CDC, 2007). In addition to contacting an ASO, people who are HIV+ can find support and connect with others who are HIV+ in various ways as recommended by the CDC (2007):

- Contact a local hospital, church, or American Red Cross chapter for referrals.
- Read HIV newsletters or magazines.
- Join support groups or Internet forums.
- Volunteer to help others with HIV.
- Be an HIV educator or public speaker, or work on a newsletter.
- Attend social events to meet other people who have HIV.

REFERENCE

Centers for Disease Control and Prevention (CDC). 2007. *Living with HIV/AIDS*. Department of Health and Human Services. Public Health Service. Atlanta, GA: Centers for Disease Control and Prevention. Accessed online December 2008. http://www.cdc.gov/hiv/resources/brochures/livingwithhiv.htm.

Stigmas can also extend to family, caregivers, and other associates of a person with, or suspected of having, HIV/AIDS, thereby reducing social support systems. Even professionals involved in HIV/AIDS service and caregiving support, such as social workers or AIDS service organization (ASO) staff, sometimes report having to deal with stigma directed toward them (e.g., Lynch and Wilson, 1996).

Stigma also often leads to discrimination, even sometimes toward the entire family of HIV+ individuals. For example, early in the U.S. epidemic when the court ordered that three HIV+ hemophiliac brothers in the Ray family could attend school after being banned from doing so, an arsonist burned the Ray family home. Each of the brothers had been infected through blood products administered for their hemophilia before blood was tested for HIV. Teenager Ryan White, also an HIV+ hemophiliac as a result of receiving infected blood products, and his family also faced discrimination and had to move in search of a supportive environment. (See Appendix B for a CDC statement on the safety of the blood supply in the United States.)

In both of these cases, social action led to policies to help those with HIV/AIDS. The Rays testified before the U.S. Senate Committee on Labor and Human Resources in 1987 (Buckley, 2001). The Ricky Ray Hemophilia Relief Fund Act of 1998 subsequently allowed the government to compensate hemophiliacs who contracted AIDS between 1982 and 1987. Ryan White became a teen activist, and a federal assistance act (discussed below) now bears his name.

POLICIES THAT PROVIDE HIV/AIDS SUPPORT

Establishing policies, as discussed in Chapter 6, is the best way to change the behaviors of large numbers of people. While no policy or legislation can, in and of itself, require people to change negative attitudes that result in stigmas, policies and legislation can accomplish, however, banning discriminatory behaviors that are often based in those attitudes. They focus on the social change work that is crucial in addressing social problems. A range of U.S. policies has been established that address HIV/AIDS. At the individual and family level, these policies can ameliorate some of the problems that HIV/AIDS bring. At the societal level, they reflect a commitment to enact social change.

Antidiscrimination Policy

Several federal policies deal with HIV/AIDS discrimination. The Americans with Disabilities Act (ADA) is central to this effort. The ADA was signed into law by President George H.W. Bush on July 26, 1990. It gives federal civil rights protections for individuals with disabilities in public accommodations, employment, transportation, state and local government services, and telecommunications. People with HIV/AIDS, whether HIV+ or diagnosed with AIDS, are considered disabled and included under coverage of the Act. Individuals who experience discrimination because they have a relationship (e.g., family) or association with (e.g., roommate) an individual who is HIV+ are also protected.

Under the ADA, qualified job applicants cannot be turned down for a job or fired based on their HIV status. Qualified applicants are those who meet the skill, experience, education, or other requirements of the job and can perform the "essential duties" of the job (in other words, the core function of what the job entails). Employers may not ask job applicants about their HIV status, require an HIV test, or provide different benefits for those who are HIV+. Also, employers must make "reasonable accommodations" for qualified applicants or employees. This means that the employer must make modifications or adjustments that would allow the disabled person to work, unless the employer would experience "undue hardship" (e.g., expense or significant difficulty) in doing so. Reasonable accommodations include such things as allowing a cashier to have a sitting stool at a cash register rather than standing an entire shift, or allowing an employee to take an extended lunch break and make up the time later to accommodate medical appointments. Exceptions require that the employer demonstrate that the person's HIV status does have some bearing in a specific situation (DOJ, n.d.).

Other federal laws also pertain to HIV/AIDS discrimination. They include the Federal Rehabilitation Act of 1973, Section 104, which prohibits disability-based discrimination in programs that receive federal assistance (including higher education). The Federal Civil Rights Act of 1991 addresses intentional discrimination and unlawful harassment in the workplace. The Air Carrier Access Act of 1986 (ACAA) prohibits disability discrimination on airlines.

Legally, friends, family, partners, or caregivers cannot be discriminated against because of their relationship with someone who is HIV+. If caregivers need time off from a job and are covered by the Family Medical Leave Act (FMLA), they cannot be prohibited from using any leave they are legally entitled to for caring for someone with HIV. (Same-sex partners are not covered under the FMLA.) However, no laws require that employers make any special arrangements for caregivers of someone with HIV (ACLU, 2006b).

Cases of HIV/AIDS-related discrimination still occur. The American Civil Liberties Union (ACLU) is active in tackling these incidents when discrimination is alleged. These acts of discrimination take diverse forms. For example, in 2005, a police chief physically blocked another person from performing CPR on a gay heart-attack victim whom he falsely assumed was HIV+ (ACLU, 2006a). Also in 2005, a cosmetology student was disenrolled from training after he revealed his HIV+ status to the owner of the beauty college (ACLU, 2005). In 2007, an RV park banned an HIV+ toddler from using the swimming pool, showers, or other areas without a doctor's note (ACLU, 2007). Only in the summer of 2008, after pressure from the ACLU, did the Peace Corps agree to change its policy to terminate volunteers solely on the basic of their HIV+ status (ACLU, 2008).

Housing Assistance

The Housing Opportunities for Persons with AIDS (HOPWA) program is the only federal program dedicated to the housing needs of people with HIV/AIDS and their families. The program began in 1992 and is administered through the Department of Housing and Urban Development (HUD). It recognizes the importance of a home as a base from which to receive HIV support and care as well as the challenges those living with HIV face in locating, securing, and maintaining housing. Two-thirds (66%) of HOPWA funds assist low income people with financial assistance for rooms, rentals, and mortgage and utility payments. Funds also pay for other supportive services that help recipients maintain their housing and maintain other needed support (e.g., case management, substance abuse/treatment). The majority (91%) of these recipients have family incomes of less than $1000 a month and also use the Ryan White Care Act and other funds. More than 80% of HOPWA-assisted households maintain a stable residence (HUD, 2008). HUD is also the primary enforcer of the Fair Housing Amendments Act of 1988 that prohibits disability-based housing discrimination, including HIV/AIDS.

Economic Assistance

In the United States and elsewhere, the effort to pay for extraordinarily expensive HIV medications and the extraordinary medical costs they incurred led some HIV patients to lose their savings and even their homes. (See Chapter 3 and the related sidebars for more information on the cost of HIV medications.). When they became too sick to work, financial strains that taxed even those with good incomes and savings mounted. Those who had health insurance had costs that exceeded benefit amounts or lost coverage altogether. As the AIDS epidemic grew, the viatical industry (see Sidebar 7.2) also grew with some AIDS patients selling their life insurance policies to pay the extensive bills they were accruing while alive.

THE VIATICAL INDUSTRY

A viatical settlement is an arrangement in which the owner of a life insurance policy (the "viator") sells their policy to a third party (often through a broker) for an immediate lump-sum cash payment that is less than the amount provided in the policy's death benefit. The third party takes over payment of the policy premiums and becomes the beneficiary, receiving the death benefit when the viator dies. The viator receives cash to use while he or she is alive and the beneficiary expects to make a profit on the investment. In simplest terms, generally the shorter the viator's life after the arrangement, the greater the profit.

One result of the growing AIDS epidemic during the 1980s was a growth in the viatical industry. Before any effective treatments were available and having AIDS was still widely considered a death sentence, selling a life insurance policy became an expedient way to pay the exorbitant medical bills many AIDS patients accrued. Some AIDS patients made quick settlements, or were taken advantage of by shady brokers negotiating the details (Leonhardt, 2005). The Federal Trade Commission (FTC) even issued a special brochure to help protect those individuals considering selling their policies in viatical arrangements from potential abuses and to help them be well-informed as to the potentially complicated legal, financial, and tax consequences involved (FTC, 1998). Investors have also been defrauded by unscrupulous companies ("Betting On Death," 2001).

As new medications have continued the length and quality of life for those with AIDS, fewer are turning to viatical settlements. However, the viatical industry itself has grown dramatically. Experts advise all parties to become knowledgeable about all the potential risks and benefits before entering into any such arrangement.

REFERENCES

"Betting on Death: Insurance Settlements Intended to Help the Dying Have Short-Changed Them and Fleeced Many Investors." *Consumer Reports*. 66: 3739, 2001.
Federal Trade Commission. 1998. "Viatical Settlements: A Guide for People with Terminal Illness." Washington, D.C.: Author. Accessed online October 2008. http://library.findlaw.com/1998/May/1/126790.html.
Leonhardt, David. 2005. "Acting Like There's No Tomorrow When There May Be Many Tomorrows Left." *New York Times*. August 8. Accessed online October 2008. http://www.nytimes.com/2005/08/08/business/08consuming.html.

The Ryan White AIDS Treatment Modernization Act of 2006 is a federal program that provides HIV-related health services for those without other means (insurance or personal financial resources) to pay for the services they need. Some technical assistance, clinical training, and research on innovative models of care are also funded through the Act. The Act is a renamed and updated version of the previous groundbreaking Ryan White Comprehensive AIDS Resources Emergency (CARE) Act of 1990, which was reauthorized in 1996 and 2000 before the 2006 version was generated.

Under the Act, agencies around the country receive federal funds. They use these funds to deliver care to eligible individuals under several funding categories, called Parts. These Parts variously fund assistance to include cities and other areas that have been hard hit by HIV/AIDS; service providers that provide early interventions; medications through the AIDS Drug Assistance Program (ADAP); services for women, infants, children, and youth, as well as families of those with HIV; Special Projects of National Significance (SPNS), which provides services to underfunded populations and addresses emerging needs; training through AIDS Education and Training Centers (AETC); dental care; and funding through the Minority AIDS Initiative that evaluates and addresses the disproportionate impact of HIV/AIDS on racial and ethnic minorities. As of 2008, the Ryan White HIV/AIDS Program was funded at $2.1 billion (HRSA, n.d.).

Economic assistance is also provided internationally thorough the United States President's Emergency Plan for AIDS Relief (PEPFAR), launched by President Bush in 2003. The Tom Lantos and Henry J. Hyde United States Global Leadership Against HIV/AIDS, Tuberculosis, and Malaria Reauthorization Act of 2008 reauthorized PEPFAR and expanded support to $48 billion. More than 2.1 million people worldwide (primarily in sub-Saharan Africa) receive antiretroviral treatment through this program, a vast increase over the estimated 500,000 who were receiving treatment before the plan was initiated (PEPFAR, 2008). However, although they admit that such gains are positive, critics argue that funding directives focusing on abstinence, requiring opposition to prostitution, and failing to integrate family planning programs into HIV prevention efforts are seriously flawed.

Critics also note that, although PEPFAR requires that funded nations have a national AIDS strategy in place, the United States has no such comprehensive strategy itself. What the United States does have is a patchwork of policy responses to HIV/AIDS. Although the Clinton administration developed a policy in 1997, critics charge that it was too vague and lacked direction and timelines. The first congressional briefing on the proposal for a national AIDS strategy for the United States was held on May 20, 2008. Advocates for such a policy have since used CDC data showing that the number of new HIV infections is 40% higher than previously estimated to argue the immediacy of the need for such a strategy.

Activists such as the National AIDS Strategy group are increasingly pressing for a strategy that has clearly articulated goals, assigned responsibilities, accountability, coordinated agency involvement, adequate funding and resources, and ongoing input from a range of interested parties (National AIDS Strategy, 2008). The Obama administration has pledged support of both PEPFAR and a national HIV/AIDS strategy.

References

American Civil Liberties Union (ACLU). 2006a. "ACLU Sues West Virginia Police Chief Who Blocked Life-Saving Measures for Gay Heart Attack Victim Assumed to Be HIV Positive." March 2. ACLU Web Site. Accessed online December 2008. http://www.aclu.org/hiv/gen/24335prs20060302.html.

_____. 2007. "ACLU Tells Alabama RV Park to Stop Discriminating against People with HIV." July 16. ACLU Web site. Accessed online December 2008. http://www.aclu.org/hiv/discrim/30572prs20070716.html.

_____. 2005. "Dugas—Arkansas Board of Cosmetology." June 2. ACLU Web site. Accessed online December 2008. http://www.aclu.org/hiv/discrim/11556res20050602.html.

_____. 2006b. "HIV & Civil Rights: Know Your Rights in the Workplace." ACLU Web site. Accessed online December 2008. http://www.aclu.org/hiv/discrim/27464res20061121.html.

_____. 2008. "Peace Corps Agrees to Stop Discriminating against Volunteers with HIV." July 30. ACLU Web site. Accessed online December 2008. http://www.aclu.org/hiv/discrim/36210prs20080730.html.

"ASO Spotlight: In This Together." 2007. *HIV Positive*. June/July: 22–24.

Buckley, Stephen. 2001. "AIDS in America: 20 Years Later. Slow Change of Heart Series: Slow Change of Heart." *St. Petersburg Times*. September 2, 1A.

Health Resources and Services Administration (HRSA). No date. "The Ryan White HIV/AIDS Program." HRSA, Department of Health and Human Services Web Site. Accessed online December 2008. http://hab.hrsa.gov/about/.

Herek, Gregory. 1999. "AIDS and Stigma." *American Behavioral Scientist*. 42, 7:1106–1116.

Lynch, Vincent J., and Paul A. Wilson. 1996. *Caring for the HIV/AIDS Caregiver*. Dover, Massachusetts: Auburn House.

Mahajan, Anish P., Jennifer N. Sayles, Vishal A. Patel, Robert H. Remien, Sharif R. Sawires, Daniel J. Ortiz, Greg Szekeres, and Thomas J. Coates. 2008. "Stigma in the HIV/AIDS Epidemic: A Review of the Literature and Recommendations for the Way Forward." *AIDS*. 22, Suppl. 2:67–80.

National AIDS Strategy. 2008. "Frequently Asked Questions." National AIDS Strategy Web site. Accessed online December 2008. http://www.nationalaidsstrategy.org/index.php?option=com_content&task=view&id=21.

Pollak, Michael, Genevieve Paicheler, and Janine Pierret. 1992. *AIDS: A Problem for Sociological Research*. London: Sage.

United States President's Emergency Plan for AIDS Relief (PEPFAR). 2008. PEPFAR Web site. Accessed online December 2008. http://www.pepfar.gov/index.htm.

U.S. Department of Housing and Urban Development (HUD). 2008. "HIV/AIDS Housing." October 28. HUD Web site. Accessed online December 2008. http://www.hud.gov/offices/cpd/aidshousing/.

U.S. Department of Justice (DOJ). No date. "Questions and Answers: The Americans with Disabilities Act and Persons with HIV/AIDS." ADA Web site. Accessed online November 2008. http://www.ada.gov/pubs/hivqanda.txt.

CHAPTER 8

Human Rights and HIV/AIDS

In this chapter, we will

- Discuss the definition of human rights
- Discuss the relationship between human rights and economic development
- Explore how HIV/AIDS is involved in violation of human rights

Human rights have become much more of a concern among the global community in the last 20 years or so. This is perhaps due in part to more knowledge about living conditions in nonindustrialized countries. With the proliferation of the Internet, increased public reporting of events, and increased accessibility to information about human rights and measurements of human rights, awareness of human rights and their relationship to everyday life issues has increased significantly.

Although there are varying definitions human rights, the best source that specifically defines human rights is the United Nations' Universal Declaration of Human Rights (UDHR), chartered in San Francisco in 1948 (UN, 1948). The UDHR has 30 articles that identify rights that should be inherently afforded and available to all humans, regardless of location, economics, politics, religion, and so forth. As it is very difficult to ensure that all humans enjoy these rights due to the various conditions that the rights are supposed to supersede, the UDHR is unfortunately, perhaps best viewed as a statement of human ideals.

To put it simply, the UDHR attempts to define the conditions necessary for human beings to thrive. Although not necessarily based on scientific research, the conditions and principles discussed in the UDHR have proven to be the ones under which human beings have the best opportunities to truly realize all of their human potential. Knowing what humans need to thrive and being able to provide all humans with those items or conditions is the difference between human rights as a set of ideals and human rights as observable reality.

The United Nations and other international agencies collect data on the quality of life in different countries. Not too surprisingly, there is a relationship between a country's economic status, the overall quality of life experienced by the majority of citizens, and the likelihood of those citizens being able to realize a number of those human rights. Generally, those countries that are highly industrialized (e.g., the United States, European Union, Japan) are much more likely to report higher standards of living, higher quality of life for their citizens, and much greater likelihood of the majority of their citizenry to be able to fulfill their human rights. Just the inverse is true for those countries that are less industrialized and less developed; their citizens are far less likely to be able to have high standards of living, good quality of life, and thus have less likelihood of fully realizing their human rights.

These varying conditions between countries are important to understand as they have a direct impact on the prevention and treatment of HIV/AIDS within populations. As one might expect, those countries that are less industrialized have higher reported cases of HIV infection and higher reported cases of AIDS. These trends are related to human rights, but not necessarily in the way one might think they are. In some countries governments intentionally work to deny their citizenry basic human rights. Obviously, these governments are characterized by corruption, their population characterized by lack of basic necessities, and attention to prevention and treatment of HIV/AIDS is severely lacking. In many other counties, however, governments are working toward trying to increase the chances of their citizenry's fulfillment of human rights, but are unable to do so due to a consistent lack of necessary resources. It is in these latter countries that human rights are less likely to be fulfilled and HIV/AIDS continue to be a national challenge.

The United Nations has taken the lead in clarifying the relationship between human rights, countries, and people with HIV/AIDS. Their most recent publication on these issues is entitled, "International Guidelines on HIV and Human Rights," released in 2006 (UNAIDS, 2006). The report provides a thorough discussion of how human rights and HIV issues are related and establishes 12 specific guidelines for what countries should do to ensure that the human rights of those with HIV or those more vulnerable to the infection are protected. Again the ability of countries to fulfill the observation of these rights is largely determined by their level of industrialization and development. Many countries lack the infrastructure, the money to create the infrastructure, and the organizational capacity to provide for the protection of human rights in relation to HIV/AIDS. Generally, it is those countries that have been hardest hit by HIV/AIDS (in the region of Sub-Saharan Africa for example) that are most in need of the ability to guarantee observation of human rights to their citizenry. But because of the distribution of HIV/AIDS and the profound impact it has on their citizenry, they are unable to develop and sustain the organizational mechanisms necessary to ensure those rights.

Historically, there have been two populations that have been less likely than other populations to fulfill their human rights; these are women and children. There has been an unfortunate history of these two groups systematically being denied their human rights. Not all of the denial was due to a dislike of these two groups; in fact much of it has been due to profound ignorance. It is these two groups that are most at-risk today for having their human rights denied. Both groups continue to be discriminated against in various forms, and it is this systematic discrimination (which in and of itself is a violation of one of the human rights outlined in the UDHR) that makes them more vulnerable to HIV infection. To provide an example of how this works, we will focus on one of the two groups, women.

Globally, women face discrimination in many areas, but most especially in three areas: literacy, violence, and social power. Discrimination in each of these areas increases the chances of contracting HIV and makes life much more difficult for women with AIDS or for women who care for others that have AIDS.

Although the global average of literacy (as defined by the percent of the population 15 and over that can read and write) is 82%; when considering gender, only 77% of women in the world are considered to be literate, as compared to 87% of men. Furthermore, two-thirds of all illiterate persons in the world are women (CIA, 2008).

For those of us living in highly industrialized countries like the United States, it might be hard to imagine how significantly the inability to read and write can impact one's life. In the United States, we take reading and writing for granted (the literacy average in the United States for both men and women is 99%; CIA, 2008). People who cannot read and write are at a severe disadvantage when it comes to finding jobs, staying on jobs, learning about new opportunities, and seizing new opportunities. Illiterate women face all of these challenges; if they or someone they care for has HIV/AIDS, they are at more of a disadvantage than a man in a similar situation. Many countries do not have free, public education like we do in the United States (generally, these are the countries with low levels of industrialization); as such, families must pay if they want their children to get an education. In many of those same countries, women are thought to not need an education, as their role is to have children, raise children, and care for all of the responsibilities of the household. It is men who are afforded the opportunity to attend school. When this occurs, women are left illiterate, uneducated, and decidedly disadvantaged.

Article 3 of the UDHR states that everyone has the right to "security of person;" in other words, everyone has a right to be safe and free from violence. As we know, violent behavior is quite common in the world; most people, despite the fact that they would say they are against the use of violence, are not surprised when hearing that violence has occurred somewhere.

In regards to women, violence, and HIV, we see more discrimination occurring. Women are oftentimes victims of violence, more often than men are. They are subjected to rape, sexual assault, human trafficking, domestic violence, female genital mutilation, and other forms of violence. In many cases, women become HIV positive as a result of the violence. Despite the fact that they are entitled to a violence- and discrimination-free life under the UDHR, this does not occur very often in practice. Women who have contracted HIV due to violence are sometimes shunned by family members, blamed for contracting the virus, and stigmatized by communities. Once again, they are subjected to systematic discrimination.

In regards to social power, many women throughout the world are not only denied education, but are also restricted to the kinds of labor that they can do. As noted above, in less industrialized, more traditional countries, more women are limited to household duties—cooking, cleaning, taking care of children, and so forth. Even in a highly industrialized country like the United States, we see women representing the vast majority of workers in "pink-collar" jobs such as daycare, elementary school teaching, clerical work, and the service industries. Traditionally, these have been their roles, and they continue to be. Although many of these roles are essential to sustaining human life, they are more often than not considered to be less important than the traditional roles that men occupy. As such, women are afforded an overall lower social status in general and do not receive the same rewards and benefits that men do. This can be seen in data collected by the United Nations on the percentage of adult women in the work force as compared to men; in all countries, there are fewer women than men employed (UNIFEM, 2008).

More evidence of how women have less social power than men lies in the distribution of women versus men in positions of political decision-making. A survey of women's representation in government positions, conducted by the United Nations, reveals that in no country do women have a major share of power. The range of women in positions of political decision-making is from 0% (Saudi Arabia, Yemen, Nauru are examples) to 49% (Rwanda) (UNIFEM, 2008).

Many people believe human rights should be guaranteed for all human beings worldwide. Unfortunately, there remains a gap between the directive of "should" and the stubborn reality of "being able to." Those countries that have had the misfortune (due to a number of factors, too many to discuss here) of not being able to industrialize and therefore not being able to compete on a global economic scale with many other countries are those less likely to be able to fulfill the requirements of human rights for all. It is also those countries that are more likely to be beset by HIV/AIDS. Ideally, all humans should have the right to those conditions and resources that encourage thriving. Our human history has been such that this has occurred differentially (especially for women and children) due to a number of different conditions. In all likelihood this differential ability to universally fulfill human rights will continue well into the future as changing resource distribution, changing social conditions, and changing traditional ways of organizing people are very difficult to do.

REFERENCES

Central Intelligence Agency (CIA). 2008. *The World Fact Book*. Washington DC: CIA. Accessed online November 2008. https://www.cia.gov/library/publications/the-world-factbook/geos/us.html.

Joint United Nations Programme on HIV/AIDS (UNAIDS). 2006. *International Guidelines on HIV/AIDS and Human Rights: 2006 Consolidated Version*. Geneva, Switzerland: UNAIDS.

United Nations (UN). 1948. *Universal Declaration of Human Rights*. New York: United Nations. Accessed online November 2008. http://www.udhr.org/UDHR/default.htm.

United Nations Development Fund for Women (UNIFEM). 2008. *Who Answers to Women? Gender and Accountability*. New York: UNIFEM.

CHAPTER 9

Popular Culture and HIV/AIDS

In this chapter, we will look at how HIV and AIDS are portrayed in various forms of popular culture, specifically

- HIV/AIDS in the visual arts
- HIV/AIDS in music
- HIV/AIDS in television and film

In the United States, the first popular press article on HIV/AIDS appeared in *The New York Times*. In July 1981, the newspaper reported on cases of a "Rare Cancer Seen in 41 Homosexuals" that had been documented that summer by the CDC (Altman, 1981). That report was the first that Americans outside of a few medical professionals had heard of what would come to be known as AIDS.

Since then, HIV and AIDS have become ingrained throughout popular culture. Popular culture, sometimes also called mass culture, refers to "cultural patterns that are widespread among a society's population" (Macionis, 2007) or among the masses. It is the lens through which many people understand and frame issues. For example, rumors, urban legends, and outright hoaxes have long fueled widespread public fears about HIV/AIDS. (See the sidebar on "Urban Legends and HIV/AIDS" and the accompanying CDC statement on "Rumors, Myths, and Hoaxes" in Appendix B.) However, in countries around the world, elements of popular culture are now used to "mainstream" and destigmatize HIV/AIDS, promote HIV/AIDS awareness and educational efforts, human rights, and social justice. A variety of formats are used, including DVDs, music videos, poster ad campaigns, television, radio, newspapers, billboards,

URBAN LEGENDS AND HIV/AIDS

One way that HIV and AIDS have become a part of our popular culture is through urban legends. Urban legends are realistic but untrue stories that recount some alleged recent event, entertainingly ironic and incredible things that have happened to some "friend of a friend." Since no one knows the source—the friend who allegedly had the experience—there is no way to verify the legitimacy of the story. Although urban legends may sound incredible, they are typically stories about things that sound at least somewhat plausible and are great for retelling. They thrive on ambiguity and the idea that the events of the story "could" have happened.

Numerous urban legends have been and continue to be circulated about HIV and AIDS. This was especially true early in the epidemic before researchers knew much about what caused AIDS and how it was transmitted, and before there were any effective medicines to treat HIV. In some HIV/AIDS urban legends, HIV was intentionally transmitted in nonsexual ways, often through infected needles allegedly left in gas pump handles, coin returns on public telephones or drink machines, and other places. Although there have been a few documented cases of an HIV+ person purposely infecting an unsuspecting person (e.g., see the summary examples given in Mikkelson, 2006, and Stine, 2008), the urban legends about needles became so prevalent that the CDC responded to the question, "Are These Stories True?" The CDC has since had to update their original answer, adding in other items. (See the primary source document "Rumors, Myths, and Hoaxes" in Appendix B.)

REFERENCES

Mikkelson, Barbara. 2006. "AIDS Mary." Urban Legends Reference Pages at snopes.com. Accessed online September 2008. http://www.snopes.com/horrors/madmen/aidsmary.asp.
Stine, Gerald J. 2008. *AIDS Update 2008*. Boston: McGraw-Hill: 209–212.

film, and literature. The portrayal of HIV/AIDS in several of these facets of popular culture are highlighted in this chapter. Chapter 4 discusses the use of popular culture in HIV/AIDS prevention and education campaigns globally.

THE ARTS AND HIV/AIDS

The arts community was hard hit from the early days of the AIDS pandemic. As a result, HIV/AIDS has long been the focus of various arts projects and members of the arts community have a long history of HIV/AIDS advocacy.

Visual Arts

Images of plague and disease have been recorded in visual arts throughout history. Artists have not only depicted the effects of physical afflictions and the social circumstances surrounding disease and illness, they have even shaped our perceptions of these concepts (Fox and Karp, 1988). The same is true for the modern pandemic of HIV/AIDS by artists working in photography, poster campaigns, and visual arts created in an array of other media.

A series of photos by Alon Reininger published in the popular *Life* magazine in 1986 brought the early AIDS pandemic powerfully and visually into the homes of mainstream America. One photograph of AIDS patient Ken Meeks showed him emaciated, seated in a wheelchair wearing a hospital gown, with visible lesions on his arms; Meeks' caregiver was in the background. Taken just three days before Meeks' death, the photo received a World Press Photo award (Garcia-Guzman, 2006).

In 1988, "Visual AIDS" was formed to use the arts to promote awareness of HIV/AIDS and to support artists with HIV/AIDS. The premiere exhibition included approximately 150 posters from 28 countries. The organizer of the exhibition noted:

> AIDS posters are among the more transient representations of the epidemic, and as such, are particularly valuable in showing that the disease is anything but an immutable set of biomedical or historical "facts" existing apart from its social constructions. (Miller, 1992: 209)

In December 1989, the first "Day With(out) Art" brought together eight hundred arts and advocacy groups to fight HIV/AIDS. Museums closed for the day and staff volunteered at AIDS services, or special exhibitions focusing on AIDS were hosted. The annual event has since expanded to include participation by several thousand organizations worldwide. Programs now showcase AIDS-related art rather than closing museums (Visual AIDS, n.d.).

The Estate Project was formed in 1991 in response to "the unprecedented impact of AIDS on American culture." Initiated by the Alliance for the Arts, the organization's mission is to provide practical estate planning advice to all artists, especially those living with HIV/AIDS; to document and offset the immense loss wrought by AIDS in all artistic disciplines; [and] to preserve the cultural legacy of the AIDS crisis so that future generations can enjoy, study, and engage artworks as aesthetic achievements and historical documents. (Bourscheidt, n.d.)

On December 1, 2003, the Estate Project launched the National Registry of Artists with AIDS. The Registry is an ongoing project that is "simultaneously a memorial to artists lost to AIDS, a tool for researchers and students, and a gateway to some of the most interesting and important cultural expression of the last 20 years" ("National Registry," n.d.).

Artist Frank Moore was involved in the creation of Visual AIDS, the AIDS ribbon (see sidebar below), and the Estate Project. He died in 2002 after being HIV+ for almost two decades. His surrealist artwork dealt with his own experiences with the virus. Other visual artists well-known for their HIV/AIDS-themed artwork include photographer Max Greenberg, who focuses on New York City scenes; Sue Coe for artwork including etches of AIDS patients; and artist/psychiatrist Dr. Eric Avery, whose art addresses a variety of social responses to issues, including HIV/AIDS.

A SYMBOL FOR HIV/AIDS

The Visual AIDS Arts Caucus created the "Red Ribbon Project" as a visual symbol of AIDS in 1991. Actor Jeremy Irons wore the ribbon at that year's Tony Awards. Yellow ribbons were popular at the time as s symbol of support for U.S. soldiers engaged in the Gulf War, and inspired the use of a ribbon to symbolize support of those infected and affected by HIV/AIDS. The color red was selected because of its "connection to blood and the idea of passion—not only anger, but love, like a valentine" (Visual AIDS Web site, n.d.). Using colorful ribbons, and more recently silicone wrist bracelets, to represent support for various causes has now become a widely recognized cultural symbol. Other causes (including alcohol/anti–drunk-driving awareness, heart disease, and stroke) now also claim the color red as their symbol.

REFERENCE

"About Visual AIDS." No date. Visual AIDS Homepage. The Body Website. Accessed online October 2008. http://www.thebody.com/visualaids/about.html.

Robert Farber, whose artwork focused on HIV/AIDS after he tested positive for HIV in 1989, created large mixed media works that took a more global and even historical perspective (Wessner, n.d.).

Music

Musicians have also given much attention to HIV/AIDS. One way they have addressed the issue is incorporating AIDS into song lyrics. Examples include Salt-N-Peppa's "Let's Talk about AIDS" (1989), Billy Joel's "We Didn't Start the Fire" (1989), Jacqui Naylor's "I Remember You" (2002), Outkast's "Roses" (2004), and the irreverent "Everyone Has AIDS" from the *Team America* soundtrack (2004) (Wessner, n.d.). The Broadway musical *Rent,* based on Giacomo Puccini's opera *La Bohème*, prominently works HIV/AIDS into its storyline about struggling young artists and musicians in New York's East Village. The show ran for 12 years on Broadway, and garnered awards including a Pulitzer Prize in Drama and a Tony Award. A movie version of *Rent* was released in 2005 to critical acclaim.

Individual musicians have also increasingly taken on the cause of fighting HIV/AIDS. Among the best known is Irish rock star Bono of the band U2. Together with Bobby Shriver, Bono established (PRODUCT) RED, a business model through which corporate brands produce RED branded products, with a portion of their sales going to the Global Fund to Fight HIV/AIDS in Africa. American singer Alicia Keys is a cofounder of and global ambassador for the Keep a Child Alive Organization that focuses on providing antiretroviral treatment in Africa. (Other global ambassadors are fashion models Iman and Padma Lakshmi.) British musician Elton John started the Elton John AIDS Foundation (EJAF) in 1992, which supports HIV/AIDS projects in the Americas and Caribbean. Elton John has long been associated with fighting HIV/AIDS. His "The Last Song" (1992), about a father and son reconciling, is used in the closing montage of the film version of *And the Band Played On*, which (as discussed below) portrays the early years of the epidemic in the United States.

The music industry has also organized to fight HIV/AIDS. Concerts began appearing on television during the late 1980s that raised awareness of HIV/AIDS (Hall, 1998) and continue not only to raise awareness, but also to conduct fundraising and encourage HIV testing. LIFEbeat, a music industry organization formed in 1992, has long focused on youth HIV/AIDS prevention and sponsors a range of innovative efforts that involve numerous musical artists from a variety of musical genres. In 2008, the popular musical competition *American Idol* gave $10 million to the Global Fund to Fight AIDS, Tuberculosis, and Malaria, raised through a special "Idol Gives Back" episode (the Global Fund, 2008).

Film and Television

Television is ubiquitous in the United States. Not only are televisions increasingly available in public venues ranging from airports to buses, "the average American home now has more television sets than people," and televisions are turned on an average of more than eight hours a day ("Average Home," 2006). Television and film have become common vehicles with which to engage popular culture on the topic of HIV/AIDS.

Film. Before the mainstream commercial film industry tackled HIV/AIDS, activists tackled the emerging epidemic through films and video. The first few of these films appeared in 1984 in Britain, but it was 1987 and later that the use of this media grew as activism increased. Included in these efforts in the United States was the Gay Men's Health Crisis (GMHC) that broadcast cable access shows as early as December 1984 and began a regular feature on "Living with AIDS" in 1987. The advocacy group ACT/UP-New York was also involved in making videos by 1989. These activist-produced videos focused on those living with HIV/AIDS, painting a more socially complex and broader picture than the mainstream media's common depictions at the time of dying white gay men, children, or other "innocent" victims of the epidemic, and racial and ethnic minority infected drug abusers (Hubbard, 2000).

Films on HIV/AIDS targeting gay and lesbian audiences also appeared during the 1980s, including *Danny, A Death in the Family,* and *A Virus Has No Morals*. In 1990, *Longtime Companion* opened in limited release, advertised as the first mainstream feature film dealing "honestly" with AIDS from a gay perspective (Beaty, 1992: 112). Actor Bruce Davison earned an Oscar nomination portraying a man who watched his lover die of AIDS.

The first made-for-television films also appeared in the 1980s, starting with *An Early Frost* (1985), a feature that focused on family strength in the story of a gay lawyer with AIDS (Harty, 1998). Several notable films aired on cable rather than network television—for example, *Common Threads: Stories from the Quilt* (1989), a film that won an Oscar for Best Documentary. As the name suggests, the film recounts stories of those memorialized in the AIDS Memorial Quilt (see sidebar). HBO also aired *And the Band Played On* in 1993, based on Randy Shilts's book by the same name that chronicles the early years of the epidemic in the United States. The politics of those early years were so contentious that the

---

THE AIDS MEMORIAL QUILT

The AIDS Memorial Quilt is a project that began in San Francisco, California. Gay-rights activist Cleve Jones teamed with some friends to memorialize those who had died of AIDS by making quilt panels in their memory. The first panel was created by Jones in 1986 in memory of his friend Marvin Feldman. The NAMES Project Foundation that oversees the quilt was formally organized by Jones, his friend Mike Smith, and others in June 1987. Since that time, the AIDS Memorial Quilt has grown to be the largest community art project in the world. It was nominated for the Nobel Peace Prize in 1989.

Individual panels of the quilt are each 3 by 6 feet. They usually include the name of the person memorialized. Otherwise, they are diverse and personal. Some include pictures or other items that represent the person's life, talents, or interests. Items incorporated into the panels include car keys, Barbie dolls, bubble wrap, merit badges, records, uniforms, and more. Panels are sewn, appliquéd, stenciled, and even painted. For display, panels are sewn together into blocks measuring 12 by 12 feet.

The quilt was displayed for the first time on the National Mall in Washington DC on October 11, 1987, during the National March on Washington for Lesbian and Gay Rights. The quilt then went on a four-month tour of major U.S. cities. At that time, it included 1,920 panels. By the end of 2008, the quilt had grown to include more than 44,000 individual panels from 35 countries in addition to the United States, sewn together into almost 6,000 blocks. The size of the entire quilt is 1,293,300 square feet, and it weighs more than 54 tons. Quilt displays have had more than 18 million visitors and raised more than $4 million in funds for direct services to benefit people with AIDS. Panels are still being added.

REFERENCE

The NAMES Foundation/AIDS Memorial Quilt Web site. Accessed online December 2008. http://www.aidsquilt.org.

---

star-studded movie took several years to make, required several rewrites and compromises in content, and has been accused by various critics of offering only a watered-down version of the events it chronicles. HBO also aired *Angels in America* (2003), an adaptation of the Tony Kushner play by the same name that had been awarded a Pulitzer Prize in Drama

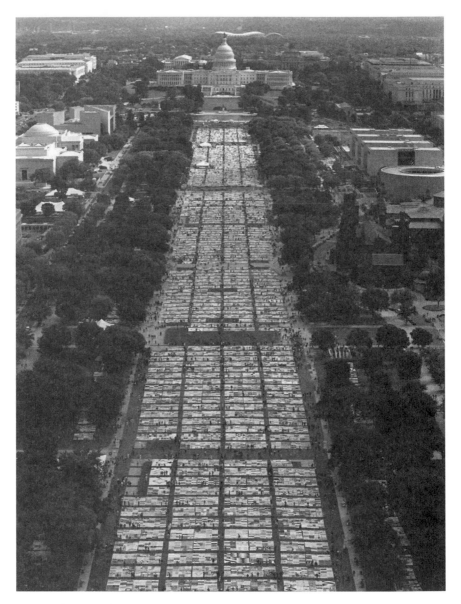

Figure 9.1 A view from the Washington Monument in 1996 shows the huge AIDS Quilt lying on the ground, stretching from the monument to the U.S. Capitol. The quilt was created in memory of those who have died from AIDS. (AP Photo/Ron Edmonds.)

and a Tony Award. Also set amidst the political controversies surrounding HIV/AIDS in the 1980s, the storyline follows the relationship of two gay couples.

Amid much press, HIV/AIDS entered the major mainstream Hollywood film industry in *Philadelphia,* released in 1993. Tom Hanks won an Academy Award as best actor for his portrayal of an attorney dying of AIDS who was locked in a discrimination lawsuit against his law firm. Hanks was seen by many commentators as taking a career risk with the role. However, some in the gay community were critical, arguing that the film de-emphasized homosexuality and failed to develop a multidimensional character, a criticism that continued at least throughout the decade (Harty, 1998). More recently, mainstream films have begun to portray more developed characters, and characters other than gay, white males. For example, the title character's love interest in *Forrest Gump* (1994) likely died of AIDS. *Boys on the Side* (1995) featured a heterosexual woman with AIDS, befriending other women on a cross-country trip.

Internationally, in 2004, India's Bollywood film industry released the first Hindi-language film *Phir Milenge* ("We Will Meet Again") dealing with HIV/AIDS. Starring Salman Khan, a well-known star in India, the film echoes *Philadelphia.* Also in 2004, the South African film *Yesterday* tells the story of an HIV+ mother. This first ever feature-length Zulu film was nominated for an Academy Award.

Television. Media messages across the television networks, including youth-oriented television programming and product advertising, are filled with sexual images. Together, these messages are a form of education for youth (a particularly vulnerable population for HIV/AIDS, as discussed in Chapter 11) about sexuality: what is accepted, expected, valued, fun, normal, and "cool." They are also often unrealistic. For example, sexual behavior on television is pervasive yet regularly depicted as having few consequences (Kunkel, Eyal, Finnerty, Biely, and Donnerstein, 2005).

Some television programming, however, has specifically targeted youth with factual information about HIV/AIDS. Some of the youth-oriented programs that have addressed HIV/AIDS have featured young people talking about or living with AIDS, such as the PBS edition of *3-2-1 Contact* that used interviews with teen AIDS activist Ryan White to tell his story (Hall, 1998). Earvin "Magic" Johnson appeared on the children's network Nickelodeon and with other celebrities including Arsenio Hall in *Time Out: The Truth About HIV, AIDS, and You* (1992). In 2002, Kami, an HIV+ character, joined the cast of the South African version of *Sesame Street.*

The MTV network that focuses on the teen and young adult market even created an AIDS celebrity, Pedro Zamora, through its programming. Zamora appeared on the 1994 season of *The Real World: San Francisco*, the third season of MTV's *Real World* series which revolves the relationships of a handful of strangers selected to be housemates. Zamora was an openly gay, HIV+, 22-year-old Cuban-born AIDS educator and activist. He had previously been featured in a *Wall Street Journal* article and interviewed by Oprah Winfrey and others, as well as testifying before Congress about HIV/AIDS education. Zamora was shown throughout the series' season educating his housemates and others about HIV/AIDS. He even exchanged rings on the show with fellow AIDS educator Sean Sasser (although the same-sex marriage was not recognized by the state of California). Zamora died days after the final episode was taped. By that time, his celebrity status had been established in popular culture. He was recognized by President Clinton for his work as an educator and activist, as well as the establishment of AIDS organizations in his name.

On daytime television, several serials (i.e., "soaps") have incorporated HIV into storylines since the late 1980s, with *General Hospital* being the first to use an HIV+ actor to portray an HIV+ character (Hall, 1998). Daytime talk show hosts have also tackled HIV/AIDS, using tactics ranging from educational efforts to the sensational. For example, several hosts, including the well-known Oprah Winfrey and Montel Williams participated in a "Day of Compassion" on June 21, 1995. The previous month, a college student had received the results of his HIV tests live on an episode of *Charles Perez* (Hall, 1998).

During evening programming, television has provided "consistent inclusion, if uneven portrayals, of AIDS" since the early days of the epidemic (Hall, 1998). In 1986, *Hill Street Blues* became the first crime series to include HIV/AIDS. Several other crime series have since incorporated HIV/AIDS into storylines, sometimes criticized by HIV/AIDS advocates as too often offering a deviant portrayal of the HIV+ character. Other popular shows, including situation comedies, dramas, and prime time serials, have integrated HIV/AIDS into storylines.

As might be expected, however, it was a medical drama that was the first evening television series to address HIV/AIDS. In 1983, the medical serial drama *St. Elsewhere,* broadcast on NBC, was the first of these programs to include AIDS in a storyline. The HIV+ character left the show. A decade later, NBC's medical drama *ER* had a several-episode storyline involving an HIV+ character depicted as living, rather than dying, with the infection. Prompted by the CDC, *ER* producers also placed a condom poster on the set to air an AIDS message. The severity of the AIDS epidemic has even compelled the CDC to partner with Hollywood in AIDS prevention efforts to provide accurate information on shows such as the popular Fox network medical drama *House* and in researching the impact of content on audience knowledge and perception (Sternberg, 2006). As discussed in Chapter 4, television soap operas and dramas, as well as feature-length films, are increasingly being utilized in global HIV/AIDS education and prevention efforts.

REFERENCES

Altman, Lawrence K. 1981. "Rare Cancer Seen in 41 Homosexuals." *New York Times*. July 3. Accessed online September 2008. http://www.nytimes.com/1981/07/03/health/03AIDS.html.

"Average Home Today Has More TVs than People." 2006. *USA Today*. September 21. Accessed online September 2008. http://www.usatoday.com/life/television/news/2006-09-21-homes-tv_x.htm.

Beaty, Bart. 1992. "The Syndrome is the System: A Political Reading of 'Longtime Companion'." In *Fluid Exchanges*. James Miller, ed. Toronto: University of Toronto: 111–121.

Bourscheidt, Randall. No date. "Mission." The Estate Project for Artists with AIDS. Alliance for the Arts Web site. Accessed online October 2008. http://www.artistswithaids.org/mission/index.html.

Garcia-Guzman, Miguel. 2006. "Giving AIDS a Human Face by Alon Reininger." Exposure Compensation Web site. Accessed online October 2008. http://exposurecompensation.com/2006/12/20/giving-aids-a-human-face-by-alon-reininger/.

"The Global Fund Welcomes Contribution from *Idol Gives Back*." 2008. November 14. The global Fund to Fight AIDS, Tuberculosis, and Malaria Website. Accessed online November 2008. http://www.theglobalfund.org/en/media_center/press/pr_081114.asp.

Hall, William Eiler. 1998. "Television Programming." In *The Encyclopedia of AIDS: A Social, Political, Cultural, and Scientific Record of the HIV Epidemic*. Raymond A. Smith, ed. New York: Routledge. Accessed online October 2008. http://www.thebody.com/content/art14041.html.

Harty, Kevin J. 1998. "Film." In *The Encyclopedia of AIDS: A Social, Political, Cultural, and Scientific Record of the HIV Epidemic*. Raymond A. Smith, ed. New York: Routledge. Accessed online October 2008. http://www.thebody.com/content/art14020.html.

Hubbard, Jim. 2000. "Fever in the Archive: AIDS Activist Video." Solomon R. Guggenheim Museum, New York. Reproduced on the Artists With AIDS Web site. Accessed online September 2008. http://www.artistswithaids.org/artery/centerpieces/centerpieces_hubbard.html.

Kunkel, Dale, Keren Eyal, Keli Finnerty, Erica Biely, and Edward Donnerstein. 2005. *Sex on TV 2005*. November. Menlo Park, CA: The Kaiser Family Foundation. Accessed online September 2008. http://www.kff.org/entmedia/upload/Sex-on-TV-4-Full-Report.pdf.

Macionis, John J. 2007. *Society: The Basics*. Upper Saddle River, NJ: Pearson/Prentice Hall.

Miller, James. 1992. "Criticism as Activism." In *Fluid Exchanges*. James Miller, ed. Toronto: University of Toronto: 185–214.

"National Registry of Artists with AIDS." No date. The Estate Project for Artists with AIDS Web site. Accessed online November 2008. http://www.artistswithaids.org/national/index.html.

Sternberg, Steve. 2006. "AIDS Drives Plots on TV." *USA Today*. August 7. Accessed online September 2008. http://www.usatoday.com/life/television/news/2006-08-07-aids-on-tv_x.htm.

"Visual AIDS Day With(out) Art." No date. Visual AIDS Homepage. The Body Web site. Accessed online October 2008. http://www.thebody.com/visualaids/dwa/dwa2006.html.

Wessner, David. No date. "HIV/AIDS in Popular Culture" Timeline. Davidson College, David Wenner Web site. Accessed online October 2008. http://www.bio.davidson.edu/projects/aidspopculture/.

CHAPTER 10

Pediatric HIV/AIDS

In this chapter, we will discuss

- Children and HIV infection
- The prevalence of HIV infection among children
- Prevention of HIV infection of children

It would seem that in the HIV/AIDS story, there is no one untouched. The story includes those who suffer with HIV infection, those who struggle with AIDS, those who love and care for these individuals; one would hope that at least one population would remain untouched. Unfortunately, this is not the case. Even those who are the most innocent have been affected. Aside from the hundreds of thousands of children who have lost mothers, fathers, and other caregivers to HIV/AIDS, there are those children who suffer directly from being HIV positive or having AIDS. Infection at infancy exacts a terrible toll on children. The WHO estimates that 30% of those infected at birth will die within one year, 50% within 2 years (UNICEF, 2008). Perhaps the most tragic aspect of their condition is that they had nothing to do with it. They were not active partners in the infection process, that is, they didn't use drugs, didn't have unprotected sexual contact, and didn't put themselves at risk in any way. They suffer nevertheless. We will look at how they become infected, how prevalent HIV infection is among children, and how infection can be prevented.

CHILDREN AND HIV INFECTION

Sadly, many children can be at risk of HIV infection before they are even born. If a mother is HIV positive, the virus is such that it can be transmitted during pregnancy, while the mother is in labor or even during delivery

(WHO, 2008a). The CDC reports that up to 25% of HIV positive women who give birth in the United States are unaware of their status (CDC, 2008b). The WHO reports that transmission during pregnancy or delivery accounts for 15% to 25% of childhood infection cases (WHO, 2008b). After birth, HIV can be transmitted through the simple act of breastfeeding; here the WHO reports that 5% to 20% of additional cases of childhood infection come through breastfeeding (WHO, 2008b). In addition, the longer a mother breastfeeds her infant, the greater is the likelihood of HIV transmission. As expected, generally those countries with higher HIV infection rates for women also have higher rates of HIV infection in children (UNICEF, 2006); typically, these are countries with far less access to medical care, fewer opportunities for adequate maternal health practices, and lower likelihoods of having nutritional needs met. Breastfeeding is much more common in these regions than in highly industrialized countries like the United States. These impoverished conditions oftentimes result in HIV-positive mothers having to choose the "lesser of two evils" because even though breastfeeding their children could transmit the virus, not breastfeeding their children has equally hazardous consequences, as explained below.

The WHO recommends breastfeeding for all infants from birth to six months, then supplementation of other food sources in addition to breast milk for up to and possibly beyond two years of age (WHO, 2008b). Despite the fact that there is a likelihood of HIV transmission through breastfeeding, the WHO still recommends that HIV positive mothers breastfeed their children for the first six months of life, as in many countries the risk of HIV infection outweighs the risk of infant mortality due to other factors such as disease, malnutrition, and other factors (WHO, 2008a). They recommend against breastfeeding if alternative feeding methods are available, affordable, and safe for the infant (WHO, 2008b). To ascertain what would be best for the infant of an HIV-infected mother, they also recommend counseling by an HIV-educated health professional.

Children also become infected through blood transfusions, violence, sexual assault, and some traditional practices such as scarification (UNAIDS, 2008). These are far less typical means of transmission than through maternal contact, which is estimated to represent 90% of childhood cases of HIV/AIDS, however (UNAIDS, 2008).

THE PREVALENCE OF HIV INFECTION AMONG CHILDREN

Data from the UN reveals that the number of children worldwide who are living with HIV/AIDS has been increasing steadily since 1990. In 1990 the estimate was between 250,000 and 500,000, and in 2007, these estimates had increased to between 2.1 and 2.3 million (UNAIDS, 2008). New infections among children have fortunately waned. In 1990, between 150,000 to 250,000 children had new infections. That number peaked in 2000, with estimates between 450,000 and 510,000. But in 2007, the estimates fell to 380,000 to 405,000 (UNAIDS, 2008). Child deaths due to AIDS have followed a similar trajectory, with low estimates of 90,000 in 1990, to highs of 380,000 in 2001, and again falling to under 300,000 in 2007 (UNAIDS, 2008). In keeping with these data the WHO estimated that 2.1 million children worldwide were living with HIV/AIDS in 2007 and of those, 2 million (95%) alone were living in Sub-Saharan Africa (WHO, 2008c).

The CDC has been tracking the estimated number of AIDS cases that resulted from maternal transmission in the United States since 1985 with the most recent data collection ending in 2006. In 1985, the estimate was less than 200 cases resulting from maternal transmission. The number of cases peaked at the end of 1992 with a high of over 800, and in 2006, the number of cases had been estimated at less than 100 (CDC, 2008a). These data indicate the spread of HIV infection due to lack of knowledge about transmission methods and less effective medications has been stemmed due to increased awareness of HIV/AIDS and much improved treatments for HIV and AIDS. The most recent data from the CDC on children and HIV indicate that in 2005, approximately 142 children received HIV from their mothers. Over 6,000 who had received the virus from their mothers were living with HIV/AIDS, and of those, 66% were African-American. Additionally, 46 children and young adults were estimated to have died due to AIDS (CDC, 2008b).

PREVENTION OF HIV INFECTION IN CHILDREN

Prevention of HIV/AIDS in children begins with the prevention of HIV/AIDS for their mothers. As we have noted, it is estimated that 90% of children become infected through maternal transmission (during pregnancy, labor, or breastfeeding). Obviously, if a mother is not HIV positive, there is no infection for her to pass on to her children. This is one more reason for continued HIV/AIDS education worldwide; prevention of one infection might be saving more than just one life.

If, however, mothers are HIV infected, there are other options available to decrease the likelihood of transmission to their children. The ability to access and utilize these additional prevention methods vary, largely due to the economic status of the country; those that are categorized as low-income (much of Africa, parts of Southeast Asia, etc.) are less likely to be able to employ these due to a lack of necessary resources. These resources include not only money for various therapies, but also knowledge, information, and skills.

In many countries (those low-income countries noted above, in particular), access to adequate prenatal and postnatal care is severely lacking. Both mother and infant have essential nutritional, safety, and attentional needs that should be met for the best health outcomes (regardless of HIV stats), but due to many infrastructural shortcomings in these countries, they are not accessible. Hence, one method of prevention is to as much as possible provide mothers and infants with the opportunities for these needs to be met and healthier outcomes to be realized. These prevention efforts, of course, require vast resources to fulfill, thus their difficulty in developing, low-income countries.

As noted above, despite the fact that breast milk can contain HIV, exclusive breast-feeding of infants for the first six months has demonstrated a decreased likelihood of infection versus nonexclusive breast-feeding (use of supplements in addition to breast milk) during this same time period (UNICEF, 2008). As such, this is one way to decrease the risk of HIV transmission for those who are unable to utilize exclusive supplementation. For many, this provides the best opportunity to live longer, even though the length of those lives may still be cut short due to HIV/AIDS.

Lastly, both mothers and infants should also receive antiretroviral prophylaxis, early antiretroviral therapies, consistent health monitoring, regular HIV testing, counseling, support, and other interventions to slow the progression of the infection (UNICEF, 2008). Again, the ability of mothers to take advantage of these interventions varies by geographic location.

As we know, not all people are born into ideal living conditions. Those that are fortunate to live in high-income countries generally have far fewer barriers and challenges to overcome when moving through life. Tragically, there are those who not only are born into extremely challenging conditions, but are also born with a life-threatening virus that, if left untreated, will drastically decrease their life span. It is, of course, unfair that this occurs; many people would agree that children are born innocent, and because of that innocence, deserve only the best opportunities that can be afforded them. As we have seen, however, millions of children worldwide are born with that innocence tainted, not due to any fault of their own, simply as a result of their birth. Through continued, collaborative, concerted efforts, however, this is changing.

REFERENCES

Centers for Disease Control and Prevention (CDC). 2008a. *Estimated Number of Perinatally Acquired AIDS Cases by Year of Diagnosis, 1985–2006—United States and*

Dependent Areas. Atlanta, GA: CDC. Accessed online November 2008. http://www. cdc.gov/hiv/topics/surveillance/resources/slides/pediatric/slides/pediatrics_4.pdf.

_____. 2008b. *Pregnancy and Childbirth.* Atlanta, GA: CDC. Accessed online November 2008: http://www.cdc.gov/hiv/topics/perinatal/index.htm.

Joint United Nations Programme on AIDS (UNAIDS). 2008. *2008 Report on the Global AIDS Epidemic.* Geneva, Switzerland: UNAIDS. Accessed online November 2008. http://www.unaids.org/en/KnowledgeCentre/HIVData/GlobalReport/2008/2008_Global_report.asp.

United Nations Children's Fund (UNICEF). 2006. *The State of the World's Children 2006: Excluded and Invisible.* Geneva, Switzerland: WHO.

World Health Organization (WHO). 2008a. *HIV and Infant Feeding.* Geneva, Switzerland: WHO. Accessed online November 2008. http://www.who.int/child_adolescent_health/topics/prevention_care/child/nutrition/hivif/en/index.html.

_____. 2008b. *HIV Transmission through Breastfeeding: A Review of Available Evidence.* Geneva, Switzerland: WHO.

_____. 2008c. *Paediatric HIV and Treatment of Children Living with HIV.* Geneva, Switzerland: WHO. Accessed online November 2008. http://www.who.int/hiv/topics/paediatric/en/index.html.

World Health Organization and the United Nations Children's Fund (UNICEF). 2008. *Scale up of HIV-Related Prevention, Diagnosis, Care and Treatment for Infants and Children: A Programming Framework.* Geneva, Switzerland, WHO & UNICEF.

CHAPTER 11

HIV/AIDS among Adolescents and Young Adults

In this chapter, we will look at

- The rates of HIV/AIDS among adolescents and young adults
- The types of behaviors that put adolescents and young adults at risk for contracting HIV
- Education, prevention, testing, and treatment focusing on these age groups

For anyone born after the summer of 1981, there has always been HIV and AIDS. They have not lived without the specter of HIV and AIDS as part of the way the world is. But are HIV and AIDS a concern for adolescents and young adults? Data from the *National Survey of Teens on HIV/AIDS 2000* conducted by the Kaiser Family Foundation says yes. Over 80% of the teens surveyed said they think that AIDS is a "very serious" or "somewhat serious" problem for teens. Additionally, over half of all teens surveyed said that they are "very concerned" (34%) or "somewhat concerned" (22%) personally about becoming infected with HIV. Younger teens (those aged 12–14) were somewhat more concerned than older teens (those aged 15–17), as were sexually active teens as compared with those who were not sexually active. Reflecting trends showing disproportionate rates of HIV in African American and Hispanic communities (see Chapter 13), African American and Latino teens expressed more personal concern than whites. Sixty percent of African American teens and 44% of Latino teens, compared to only 28% of white teens, agreed they were very concerned (Kaiser Family Foundation, 2000).

Sixteen percent of teens in the survey personally knew someone who had AIDS, had died from AIDS, or had tested positive for HIV. Females, older teens, and those who were already sexually active were more likely than males, younger teens, and those who were not sexually active to know someone in one of these categories. So were African American and Latino teens as compared to whites (28%, 20%, and 14% respectively).

HIV/AIDS is increasing among adolescents and young adults. In the United States, the number of newly diagnosed cases of HIV as well as the number of persons living with AIDS among people aged 15–24 both increased from 2003 through 2006 (CDC, 2008). The number of deaths of persons with AIDS also increased for this age group during that same time frame (CDC, 2008). In 2006, almost 19,000 people aged 15–24 were living with HIV/AIDS and almost 10,000 people in this age group were known to have already died since the beginning of the pandemic (CDC, 2008).

Globally, over 10 million young people aged 15–24 are HIV+. Half of all HIV transmission occurs within this age group (Ross, Dick, and Ferguson, 2006; UNICEF, UNAIDS, and WHO, 2002). And the numbers are growing with more than 5,000 young people becoming infected daily. Sub-Saharan Africa is especially impacted by the youth AIDS crisis, with over 6 million youth already infected, followed by Asia with 2.2 million HIV+ youth. In eastern Europe and central Asia, nearly half of all HIV+ adults (600,000/1.3 million) are under age 25 (Ross, Dick, and Ferguson, 2006).

WHAT BEHAVIORS PUT TEENS AND YOUNG ADULTS AT RISK FOR HIV?

Some HIV+ teens and young adults were infected at birth or through breastfeeding and have grown up with HIV infection. However, most HIV+ teens contracted the virus through their own behavior. Adolescence is widely considered a time of sexual exploration, asserting independence, and of engaging in risky behaviors in general. Teens often do dangerous things because their age group tends to feel relatively invulnerable and be subject to peer pressure. Taking dangerous risks and making poor decisions can be compounded when youth (or those of any age group) use drugs or alcohol. Additionally, teens and young adults often lack accurate information about sexuality in general and HIV/AIDS specifically. This puts them at an increased risk for pregnancy as well as contracting sexually transmitted infections (STIs), including HIV (e.g., UNICEF, UNAIDS, and WHO, 2002). According to data from the CDC, the majority of all HIV/AIDS cases in teens are the result of sexual transmission (CDC, 2008). Rates of other sexually transmitted infections are also high among youth (Miller et al., 2004, 2005).

But how sexually active are teens? And what types of risks do they commonly take? The CDC gathers this type of information through the Youth Risk Behavior Surveillance System (YRBSS). According to YRBSS data for 2007, almost half (47.8%) of high school students across the United States reported that they have had sexual intercourse at least once. More than one third (35%) reported that they were sexually active at the time the survey was taken. Nationwide, 7.1% of these teens had engaged in sexual intercourse for the first time before they were 13 years old. Almost 15% of these high schoolers reported having had sexual intercourse with four or more persons during their lives, males more so than females (17.9% and 11.8% respectively) (Eaton et al., 2008).

These teens do not always rely on condoms for protection from pregnancy or STIs. Of all those high schoolers who were sexually active, over one third (38.5%) had not used a condom the last time they had sexual intercourse (Eaton et al., 2008). Similarly, in the *National Survey of Teens on HIV/AIDS 2000,* only 65% said that they use condoms "all the time" when they have sexual intercourse (Kaiser Family Foundation, 2000). Younger teens and those who have dropped out of school are less likely to use condoms than their peers or older counterparts (Office of the Surgeon General, 2001; UNICEF, UNAIDS, and WHO, 2002).

Almost a quarter (22.5%) of sexually active students compounded risky behaviors by using alcohol or other drugs, sometimes before engaging in sexual intercourse (Eaton, 2008). Intravenous drug use, another route of transmission for HIV, generally begins in adolescence. In the United States, 2% of high school students nationwide report having injected illegal intravenous drugs, and 3.9% have taken unprescribed steroids (including shots) (Eaton et al., 2008). Rates of drug use are even higher for those youth who have dropped out of school.

Participating in sexual activities is not always voluntary. Almost 8% (7.8%) of high school students nationwide reported that they have been physically forced to have sexual intercourse when they did not want to do so. This was more the case for females (11.3%) than for males (4.5%) (Eaton et al., 2008). Globally, sexual coercion, abuse, and trafficking have been especially implicated in the growth of AIDS with runaways and children living on the street being at special risk for HIV.

Around the world, social factors such as poverty, inequality, cultural traditions that encourage early sexual activity and devalue women by supporting non-monogamous male sexuality, violence against women, older

men having sex with much younger girls, and early marriages are responsible for increasing rates of HIV and AIDS among teens and young adults.
Young women are increasingly being infected because of this range of
factors. In sub-Saharan Africa, the infection rate for adolescent and young
adult women is three times that of men (UNAIDS, 2004). Myths and misinformation also fuel these high infection rates for females. For example,
the myths that having sexual intercourse with a virgin can cure HIV or that
younger girls will not be infected have fueled the crisis in Africa (Ross,
Dick, and Ferguson, 2006; UNICEF, UNAIDS, and WHO, 2002).

ADDRESSING HIV/AIDS AMONG TEEN AND YOUNG ADULTS

To best address HIV/AIDS among teens and young adults, it is important to start with what they know, and what they do not know about
HIV/AIDS. Data from the *National Survey of Teens on HIV/AIDS 2000*
show that American teens know some basic information about HIV and
AIDS, but want to know more (Kaiser Family Foundation, 2000). Over
90% of teens know that sharing needles and having unprotected sexual
intercourse are risk factors for HIV transmission (92% and 91% respectively). Yet, only 69% know that unprotected oral sex is also a risk factor
and even fewer (41%) know that having another sexually transmitted
infection increases the risk of HIV transmission. International data show
that perhaps as many as 80% of young women do not have basic knowledge of HIV (Ross, Dick, and Ferguson, 2006).

Many teens could also be better informed about some other basic
aspects of HIV/AIDS (Kaiser Family Foundation, 2000). While 79% of
teens know that there is no cure for AIDS, only 51% know that life-
extending drugs are available for those infected with HIV. Twenty-seven
percent think that a parents' permission is required for a person under age
18 to get an HIV test.

Education

Teens get much of their information on HIV/AIDS at school from their
teachers, school nurses, or in the classroom. Over 60% of teens in the
National Survey of Teens on HIV/AIDS 2000 say they get "a lot" and 18%
say they get "some" of their HIV/AIDS information from those sources
(Kaiser Family Foundation, 2000). Most students in the YRBSS say they
are being educated about HIV and AIDS in school (Eaton et al., 2008).
They do not, however, report this consistently throughout the United
States. Over 90% (91.7%) of students in Connecticut report having had

HIV or AIDS education. That is the highest rate of any state. Only 79% of students from Arizona said they have had HIV or AIDS education. That is the lowest percentage of any state (see Table 11.1). Additionally, only a median of 2.2 hours of HIV prevention is provided in high school courses that do require it be taught, and the percentage of states providing staff development on HIV prevention decreased from 96.1% to 84% between 2000 and 2006 (SHPPS, 2007). Chapter 4 provides more discussion on school-based education programs.

Prevention

Teens want to know more about HIV prevention and testing. In the *National Survey of Teens on HIV/AIDS 2000*, teens said they want to know more about how to protect themselves from HIV (57%), what AIDS is and how it is transmitted (48%), and how to talk with a partner (46%) or parents (40%) about HIV/AIDS. Just over one third (36%) said they want to know more about the proper way to use condoms, and 69% said that high schools should provide students with condoms if the student asks (Kaiser Family Foundation, 2000). How to correctly use a condom is, however, taught in only 38.5% of high schools in which HIV prevention is required instruction (SHPPS, 2007). Promising prevention programs have been developed specifically for adolescents and young adults who are HIV positive. These programs are designed to reduce high risk behaviors, improve healthy behaviors, and improve quality of life (Tevendale and Lightfoot, 2006).

Testing

Additionally, knowing one's own HIV status is crucial, not only in getting appropriate treatment, but in preventing transmission of the virus. Only one quarter (27%) of sexually active teens in the *National Survey of Teens on HIV/AIDS 2000* had ever been tested for HIV (Kaiser Family Foundation, 2000). Slightly less than half (48%) said that if they wanted to get tested, they are sure that they know where to go. One third (35%) had some idea where to go for testing, but 17% said they have no idea where to go for HIV testing.

Health care providers broaching the subject of HIV testing and targeted marketing campaigns aimed at encouraging youth to be tested have increased the rates of testing among this age group. The greater availability of rapid HIV testing methods that allow results within a half hour, rather than requiring a wait of days or weeks and a second visit to the testing facility, are also preferred by adolescents and young adults.

Table 11.1 Percentage of high school students who drank alcohol or used drugs before last sexual intercourse* and who were ever taught in school about acquired immunodeficiency syndrome (AIDS) or human immunodeficiency virus (HIV) infection, by sex—selected U.S. sites (CDC, Youth Risk Behavior Survey, 2007)

	Drank alcohol or used drugs before last sexual intercourse					
	Female		Male		Total	
Site	%	CI[†]	%	CI	%	CI
State Surveys						
Alaska	21.5	14.7–30.5	22.9	16.9–30.2	**22.1**	**17.0–28.2**
Arizona	20.4	15.4–26.5	35.2	29.7–41.2	**27.6**	**23.1–32.5**
Arkansas	16.5	12.0–22.3	25.3	18.5–33.6	**20.6**	**16.6–25.2**
Connecticut	22.7	17.1–29.6	33.9	28.0–40.4	**27.9**	**23.1–33.3**
Delaware	16.1	13.0–19.9	26.3	22.0–31.1	**21.6**	**18.8–24.6**
Florida	17.5	14.6–20.7	25.6	22.7–28.6	**21.8**	**19.7–24.0**
Georgia	—[‡]	—	—	—	—	—
Hawaii	21.6	16.3–28.0	—	—	**27.2**	**20.3–35.4**
Idaho	—	—	—	—	—	—
Illinois	19.7	15.4–24.8	24.9	19.9–30.5	**22.0**	**18.3–26.4**
Indiana	19.3	15.1–24.3	28.7	21.1–37.7	**23.5**	**19.1–28.7**
Iowa	16.4	13.2–20.2	19.9	13.5–28.4	**18.0**	**14.1–22.8**
Kansas	20.8	16.6–25.6	31.3	23.3–40.5	**25.9**	**20.7–31.7**
Kentucky	17.2	13.9–20.9	21.4	17.0–26.5	**19.0**	**16.1–22.3**
Maine	16.3	11.3–23.0	25.0	17.6–34.4	**20.3**	**16.7–24.5**
Maryland	—	—	—	—	—	—
Massachusetts	21.9	17.7–26.7	27.7	22.9–33.2	**24.6**	**20.7–29.0**
Michigan	21.3	17.2–26.0	25.2	19.9–31.3	**23.2**	**19.9–26.9**
Mississippi	10.7	8.5–13.5	24.0	18.6–30.4	**17.6**	**14.1–21.9**
Missouri	16.8	11.4–24.0	27.8	19.6–37.9	**21.9**	**16.3–28.9**
Montana	21.3	18.1–25.0	32.2	27.3–37.5	**26.0**	**23.0–29.1**
Nevada	18.3	13.9–23.6	24.7	19.4–30.9	**21.5**	**17.9–25.6**
New Hampshire	20.2	15.9–25.4	28.4	22.5–35.2	**24.3**	**20.1–28.9**
New Mexico	19.8	13.6–27.9	28.7	23.3–34.9	**23.7**	**19.5–28.5**
New York	19.3	14.9–24.5	26.8	21.5–32.8	**22.8**	**18.7–27.5**
North Carolina	17.4	13.2–22.6	24.3	20.2–28.9	**20.7**	**17.6–24.1**
North Dakota	26.8	20.8–33.9	29.6	23.9–35.9	**28.1**	**23.8–32.9**
Ohio	18.4	15.3–22.0	26.9	22.5–31.8	**22.5**	**19.7–25.5**
Oklahoma	17.4	12.5–23.7	30.0	22.6–38.5	**23.3**	**18.4–29.0**
Rhode Island	14.8	11.0–19.6	25.2	19.8–31.5	**20.1**	**16.3–24.5**
South Carolina	16.8	12.8–21.9	21.1	13.7–30.9	**18.8**	**13.7–25.3**
South Dakota	25.7	18.4–34.6	29.5	24.1–35.5	**27.3**	**21.6–33.9**
Tennessee	13.7	10.0–18.4	24.8	18.9–31.8	**19.4**	**15.3–24.3**
Texas	18.9	15.1–23.5	25.5	21.1–30.5	**22.2**	**19.3–25.4**
Utah	—	—	—	—	—	—
Vermont	21.9	17.8–26.7	32.8	27.4–38.8	**27.2**	**22.6–32.4**
West Virginia	20.3	16.1–25.3	23.9	17.7–31.3	**22.3**	**18.3–26.8**
Wisconsin	21.7	17.1–27.0	32.7	27.4–38.4	**26.6**	**23.1–30.5**
Wyoming	20.0	16.5–23.9	30.4	25.7–35.6	**25.0**	**21.9–28.3**

Were taught in school about AIDS or HIV infection					
Female		Male		Total	
%	CI	%	CI	%	CI
84.6	80.0–88.3	86.9	83.3–89.8	**85.8**	**83.3–88.0**
80.4	76.4–83.9	77.6	73.1–81.6	**79.0**	**75.1–82.5**
86.6	83.0–89.5	84.7	80.1–88.4	**85.6**	**82.2–88.4**
91.8	89.2–93.9	91.6	88.7–93.8	**91.7**	**89.5–93.4**
91.7	89.9–93.2	89.5	87.6–91.2	**90.4**	**89.0–91.6**
90.4	88.3–92.1	85.9	83.8–87.8	**88.0**	**86.2–89.6**
92.5	90.4–94.1	88.8	86.3–90.8	**90.6**	**88.8–92.0**
86.4	83.1–89.1	87.9	84.3–90.8	**87.1**	**84.4–89.5**
84.0	78.1–88.6	80.9	75.8–85.1	**82.2**	**77.4–86.2**
91.8	89.2–93.8	89.4	86.0–92.0	**90.6**	**88.0–92.7**
91.6	88.6–93.9	87.7	85.3–89.7	**89.3**	**87.1–91.2**
89.3	83.9–93.0	85.7	80.9–89.4	**87.5**	**83.0–90.9**
87.2	83.8–89.9	82.6	77.8–86.5	**84.8**	**81.5–87.6**
87.5	84.2–90.2	86.3	84.0–88.3	**86.8**	**84.8–88.6**
88.3	82.7–92.3	85.9	82.0–89.1	**87.1**	**84.3–89.4**
88.7	85.3–91.5	82.5	78.1–86.1	**85.3**	**82.5–87.7**
89.4	86.7–91.6	87.9	84.9–90.3	**88.5**	**86.0–90.6**
90.2	86.9–92.7	89.2	86.8–91.2	**89.6**	**87.4–91.5**
83.2	78.5–87.0	80.6	76.6–84.0	**81.7**	**78.0–84.9**
89.3	84.1–92.9	86.9	81.9–90.6	**88.0**	**83.7–91.3**
90.4	88.4–92.0	89.4	87.5–91.0	**89.7**	**88.3–91.0**
82.5	78.3–85.9	82.1	78.6–85.2	**82.3**	**79.7–84.6**
88.7	85.8–91.0	89.5	86.8–91.7	**89.0**	**87.0–90.8**
82.7	75.6–88.1	83.1	75.6–88.7	**82.7**	**75.7–88.0**
89.8	87.6–91.6	86.0	83.2–88.5	**87.8**	**85.9–89.6**
—	—	—	—	**—**	**—**
—	—	—	—	**—**	**—**
89.0	87.1–90.7	88.5	86.2–90.5	**88.8**	**87.1–90.3**
89.7	86.7–92.0	88.4	86.1–90.4	**89.0**	**86.8–90.9**
90.8	88.0–93.0	88.0	84.5–90.8	**89.4**	**87.0–91.4**
89.2	86.0–91.8	85.4	80.2–89.4	**87.1**	**84.7–89.3**
85.9	80.8–89.8	84.7	80.6–88.0	**85.3**	**81.0–88.8**
90.9	88.1–93.2	87.0	83.2–90.1	**88.9**	**86.0–91.3**
86.9	84.6–88.9	84.0	80.3–87.2	**85.5**	**82.9–87.7**
85.0	81.7–87.8	81.7	75.1–86.8	**82.9**	**78.4–86.7**
—	—	—	—	**—**	**—**
88.5	83.5–92.1	87.1	79.6–92.1	**87.8**	**81.9–91.9**
—	—	—	—	**—**	**—**
87.3	84.1–89.8	84.7	82.1–87.0	**85.7**	**83.7–87.6**

(Continued)

Table 11.1 *(Continued)*

	Drank alcohol or used drugs before last sexual intercourse					
	Female		Male		Total	
Site	%	CI	%	CI	%	CI
State Surveys						
Median	19.3	26.5	22.5	88.7	**86.3**	**87.5**
Range	10.7–		19.9–		**17.6–**	
	26.8		35.2		**28.1**	
Local Surveys						
Baltimore, MD	8.1	5.7–11.4	16.1	12.3–20.8	**12.2**	**9.7–15.3**
Boston, MA	16.0	11.9–21.3	25.6	19.9–32.1	**21.2**	**17.8–25.1**
Broward County, FL	14.0	8.2–22.9	23.5	16.5–32.4	**19.2**	**13.7–26.2**
Charlotte-Mecklenburg, NC	11.6	8.1–16.5	18.8	14.1–24.5	**15.2**	**11.8–19.3**
Chicago, IL	8.7	5.0–14.9	17.4	10.0–28.6	**12.5**	**8.1–18.7**
Dallas, TX	9.2	5.6–14.6	25.4	19.5–32.3	**17.7**	**13.9–22.3**
DeKalb County, GA	11.5	8.3–15.7	17.5	14.0–21.6	**14.6**	**12.0–17.6**
Detroit, MI	12.4	8.7–17.4	14.2	10.5–18.8	**13.5**	**10.9–16.7**
District of Columbia	14.9	11.1–19.6	20.6	15.0–27.6	**17.4**	**14.2–21.1**
Hillsborough County, FL	16.5	11.2–23.6	25.6	19.2–33.2	**20.5**	**16.3–25.3**
Houston, TX	10.5	7.5–14.6	18.8	14.1–24.7	**14.6**	**11.6–18.2**
Los Angeles, CA	14.6	9.0–22.8	23.8	16.9–32.4	**19.8**	**15.7–24.7**
Memphis, TN	7.7	4.7–12.5	16.7	12.4–22.1	**12.3**	**9.4–15.9**
Miami-Dade County, FL	15.5	11.8–19.9	23.7	19.2–28.8	**20.2**	**17.3–23.3**
Milwaukee, WI	12.8	9.5–17.2	23.9	18.4–30.5	**18.2**	**15.0–21.9**
New York City, NY	10.1	7.7–13.1	17.0	13.5–21.1	**13.4**	**11.3–15.7**
Orange County, FL	16.7	9.4–28.0	18.8	12.7–26.8	**17.5**	**11.9–25.1**
Palm Beach County, FL	21.6	15.4–29.4	29.9	24.9–35.5	**25.5**	**21.4–30.1**
Philadelphia, PA	11.5	8.2–15.8	18.4	14.5–23.1	**14.8**	**12.2–17.9**
San Bernardino, CA	17.0	11.9–23.8	21.0	15.0–28.7	**19.3**	**15.3–24.1**
San Diego, CA	14.4	9.8–20.6	27.5	20.5–36.0	**20.9**	**16.8–25.8**
San Francisco, CA	15.0	11.2–19.8	13.6	9.3–19.4	**14.4**	**11.5–17.9**
Median	13.4	19.7	17.4			
Range	7.7–		13.6–		**12.2–**	
	21.6		29.9		**25.5**	

*Among students who were currently sexually active

†95% confidence interval.

‡Not available.

Were taught in school about AIDS or HIV infection					
Female		Male		Total	
%	CI	%	CI	%	CI
80.4–92.5		77.6–91.6		79.0–91.7	
89.6	87.4–91.5	85.7	82.7–88.3	**87.7**	**85.9–89.3**
77.7	73.2–81.6	76.1	71.2–80.3	**76.9**	**73.2–80.1**
92.0	89.6–94.0	86.1	82.8–88.8	**89.0**	**87.6–90.3**
—	—	—	—	**—**	**—**
87.7	82.3–91.6	80.3	72.2–86.5	**84.1**	**79.1–88.1**
77.6	73.5–81.2	75.8	69.0–81.5	**76.7**	**73.3–79.8**
90.5	88.5–92.2	85.3	83.0–87.3	**87.8**	**86.1–89.2**
85.6	82.9–88.0	81.5	77.8–84.6	**83.7**	**81.1–85.9**
88.4	85.5–90.7	82.4	78.4–85.8	**85.7**	**83.2–87.9**
94.7	92.3–96.4	89.9	86.7–92.3	**92.3**	**90.4–93.9**
80.8	77.0–84.1	76.9	73.0–80.5	**78.7**	**75.7–81.5**
81.1	73.1–87.2	82.8	75.9–88.1	**82.1**	**75.4–87.2**
87.6	84.3–90.3	83.6	79.3–87.2	**85.7**	**83.1–88.0**
87.7	84.6–90.2	84.8	81.0–87.9	**85.9**	**82.9–88.4**
—	—	—	—	**—**	**—**
89.6	87.2–91.6	86.1	83.7–88.2	**88.0**	**86.0–89.7**
89.1	86.2–91.4	87.9	84.7–90.5	**88.5**	**86.3–90.4**
86.9	83.6–89.6	84.4	80.5–87.6	**85.6**	**82.6–88.1**
86.3	83.1–88.9	81.8	78.3–84.8	**84.4**	**81.6–86.9**
82.8	78.4–86.4	82.1	78.0–85.6	**82.5**	**78.8–85.6**
86.3	83.4–88.8	87.0	83.1–90.1	**86.5**	**83.9–88.8**
86.3	82.8–89.2	84.7	81.6–87.3	**85.5**	**82.9–87.8**
87.2		84.0		**85.6**	
77.6–94.7		75.8–89.9		**76.7–92.3**	

Table 68 in Eaton, Danice K., Laura Kann, Steve Kinchen, Shari Shanklin, James Ross, Joseph Hawkins, William A. Harris, Richard Lowry, Tim McManus, David Chyen, Connie Lim, Nancy D. Brener, and Howell Wechsler. June 6, 2008 "Youth Risk Behavior Surveillance—United States, 2007." *Morbidity and Mortality Weekly Report* (*MMWR*). 57, (SS 4):1–131. Accessed online July 2008. http://www.cdc.gov/mmwr/preview/mmwrhtml/ss5704a1.htm?s_cid=ss5704a1_e. Centers for Disease Control.

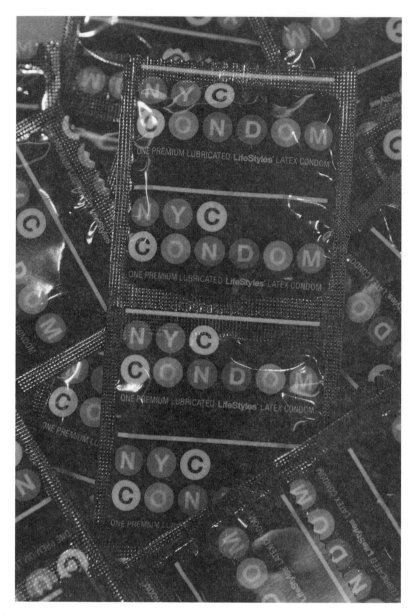

Figure 11.1 Packets of the nation's first city-themed condoms are displayed inside a Kenneth Cole store in New York after authorities unveiled the condoms—designed to mimic the look of the city's subway lines—on Valentine's Day 2007. The condoms, which have been promoted with such slogans as "New York: We've got you covered" and "NYC condoms. Get some," are part of a drive by the city's health department to increase condom use. (Courtesy AP Photo/Kathy Willens.)

Treatment

The prospect of taking drugs for life can be daunting for anyone, especially teens and young adults. Additionally, other life circumstances such as poverty, violent or abusive situations, and homelessness may seem more immediate or burdensome than taking medication as prescribed and make following a strict treatment regimen more problematic (Martinez et al., 2000; Remein et al., 2003). The few intervention strategies specifically designed and studied regarding teen adherence to Highly Active Antiretroviral Therapy (HAART) have largely relied on peer and group support, or individual counseling and have reported limited success (e.g., Rotheram-Borus et al., 2004). The HAART regimen (see Chapter 3) requires strict adherence to work well, and this has proven difficult for many people (Chesney et al., 1999). The adherence rate for this treatment is especially low for teens and young adults (e.g., Becker et al., 2002; Murphy et al., 2003). Hopefully, as treatment continues to evolve resulting in simplified regimens and adjusted dosage, teen and young adult adherence to those regimens will increase.

When treatment fails, only a small body of research addresses HIV+ teens or young adults who are facing death, and their families. Parents and youth in this situation may desire, and benefit from, sensitive supports to help them communicate, plan, and deal with the range of emotional, financial, medical, and ethical issues involved (Lyon and Pao, 2006).

REFERENCES

Alford S. 2008. *Science and Success, Second Edition: Sex Education and Other Programs That Work to Prevent Teen Pregnancy, HIV & Sexually Transmitted Infections.* Washington, D.C.: Advocates for Youth. Accessed September 2008. http://www.advocatesforyouth.org/programsthatwork/intro.htm.

Becker S.L., C.M. Dezii, B. Burtcel, H. Kawabata, S. Hodder. 2002. "Young HIV-Infected Adults Are at Greater Risk for Medication Nonadherence." *Medscape General Medicine.* 4 (3), 2002. Accessed online September 2008. http://www.medscape.com/viewarticle/438510.

Centers for Disease Control and Prevention (CDC). 1999. *CDC HIV/AIDS Prevention Research Project Compendium of HIV Prevention Interventions with Evidence of Effectiveness.* Atlanta: CDC.

_____. 1988, revised 2003. "Guidelines for Effective School Health Education to Prevent the Spread of AIDS." *Morbidity & Mortality Weekly Report Supplement.* January 29. Accessed online September 2008. http://www.cdc.gov/HealthyYouth/sexualbehaviors/guidelines/index.htm.

_____. 2008. *HIV/AIDS Surveillance Report, 2006*. Vol. 18. Atlanta: U.S. Department of
    Health and Human Services, Centers for Disease Control and Prevention. Accessed
    online July 2008. http://www.cdc.gov/hiv/topics/surveillance/resources/reports/
    2006report/pdf/2006SurveillanceReport.pdf.
Chesney, M.A., J. Ickovics, F.M. Hecht, G. Sikipa, and J. Rabkin. 1999. "Adherence: A
    Necessity for Successful HIV Combination Therapy." *AIDS*. 13, Suppl. A: S271–278.
DiClemente, Ralph J., and Richard A. Crosby. 2006. "Preventing HIV Infection in Ado-
    lescents: What Works for Uninfected Teens." In *Teenagers, HIV, and AIDS*: *Insights
    from Youths Living with the Virus*. Lyon, Maureen E., and Lawrence J. D'Angelo, eds.
    Westport, CT: Praeger:143–161.
Eaton, Danice K., Laura Kann, Steve Kinchen, Shari Shanklin, James Ross, Joseph
    Hawkins, William A. Harris, Richard Lowry, Tim McManus, David Chyen, Connie
    Lim, Nancy D. Brener, and Howell Wechsler. June 6, 2008 "Youth Risk Behavior
    Surveillance—United States, 2007." *Morbidity and Mortality Weekly Report* (*MMWR*).
    57, (SS 4):1–131. Accessed online July 2008. http://www.cdc.gov/mmwr/preview/
    mmwrhtml/ss5704a1.htm?s_cid=ss5704a1_e.
Joint United Nations Programme on HIV/AIDS (UNAIDS). 2004. *2004 Report on the
    Global AIDS Epidemic*. Geneva, Switzerland: UNAIDS. Accessed online August 2008.
    http://www.unaids.org/bangkok2004/GAR2004_html/GAR2004_00_en.htm.
Kaiser Family Foundation. 2000. *National Survey of Teens on HIV/AIDS 2000*. Menlo
    Park, CA: Kaiser Family Foundation. Accessed online September 2008.
    http://www.kff.org/youthhivstds/upload/National-Survey-of-Teens-on-HIV-AIDS.pdf.
Lyon, Maureen E., and Maryland Pao. 2006. "When All Else Fails: End-of-Life Care for
    Adolescents." In *Teenagers, HIV, and AIDS*: *Insights from Youths Living with the Virus*.
    Lyon, Maureen E., and Lawrence J. D'Angelo, eds. Westport, CT: Praeger: 215–233.
Martinez, J., D. Bell, R. Camacho, L.M. Henry-Reid, M. Bell, C. Watson, and F. Rodriguez.
    2000. "Adherence to Antiviral Drug Regimens in HIV-infected Adolescent Patients
    Engaged in Care in a Comprehensive Adolescent and Young Adult Clinic." *Journal of the
    National Medical Association*. 92, 2: 55–61.
Miller, W.C., C.A. Ford, M. Morris, M.S. Handcock. J.L. Schmitz, M.M. Hobbs, M.S.
    Cohen, K.M. Harris, and J.R. Udry. 2004. "Prevalence of Chlamydial and Gonococcal
    Infections among Young Adults in the United States." *JAMA*. 291, 18: 2229–2236.
Miller, W.C., M.M. Hobbs, C.A. Ford, M.S. Handcock, M. Morris, J.L. Schmitz, M.S.
    Cohen, K.M. Harris, and J.R. Udry. 2005. "The Prevalence of Trichomoniasis in Young
    Adults in the United States." *Sexually Transmitted Diseases*. 32, 10: 593–598.
Murphy, D.A., M. Sarr, S.J. Durako, A.B. Moscicki, C.M. Wilson, and L.R. Muenz. 2003.
    "Barriers to HAART Adherence among Human Immunodeficiency Virus-Infected
    Adolescents." *Archives of Pediatric Adolescent Medicine*. 157, 3: 249–255.
Office of the Surgeon General. July 9, 2001. *The Surgeon General's Call to Action to Pro-
    mote Sexual Health and Responsible Sexual Behavior*. Washington, D.C.: Department

of Health and Human Services. Accessed online September 2008. http://www.surgeon-general.gov/library/sexualhealth/call.htm.

Remein, R.H., A.E. Hirky, M.O. Johnson, L.S. Weinhardt, D. Whittier, and G.M. Le. 2003. "Adherence to medication treatment: A Qualitative Study of Facilitators and Barriers among a Diverse Sample of HIV+ Men and Women in Four U.S. Cities." *AIDS Behavior*. 7, 1: 61–72.

Ross, David A., Brice Dick, and Jane Ferguson, eds. 2006. *Preventing HIV/AIDS in Young People: A Systematic Review of the Evidence from Developing Countries*. UNAIDS Interagency Task Team on HIV and Young People. Geneva, Switzerland: World Health Organization. Accessed online September 2008. http://whqlibdoc.who.int/trs/WHO_TRS_938_eng.pdf.

Rotheram-Borus, M.J., J.D. Swendeman, W.S. Comulada, R.E. Weiss, M. Lee, and M. Lightfoot. 2004. "Prevention for Substance-using HIV-positive Young People: Telephone and In-Person Delivery." *Journal of Acquired Immunodeficiency Syndrome*. 37, Suppl 2: S68–77.

School Health Policies and Programs Study (SHPPS). 2007. *Journal of School Health*. 77, 8. October 2007 edition of journal devoted to comprehensive discussion of SHPPS.

Tevendale, Heather D., and Marguerite Lightfoot. 2006. "Programs that Work: Prevention for Positives." In *Teenagers, HIV, and AIDS*: *Insights from Youths Living with the Virus*. Lyon, Maureen E., and Lawrence J. D'Angelo, eds. Westport, CT: Praeger: 63–178.

Underhill, Kristen, Paul Montgomery, and Don Operario. 2007. "Sexual Abstinence Only Programmes to Prevent HIV Infection in High Income Countries: Systematic Review." *BMJ (British Medical Journal)*. 335, 7613: 248–259.

United Nations Children's Fund (UNICEF), Joint United Nations Programme on HIV/AIDS (UNAIDS), and World Health Organization (WHO). 2002. *Young People and HIV/AIDS: Opportunity in Crisis*. New York/Geneva. Accessed online September 2008. http://www.unicef.org/vietnam/Opportunity_in_Crisis.pdf.

CHAPTER 12

HIV/AIDS and Older Adults

In this chapter, we will look at

- Increasing rates of HIV/AIDS among adults aged 50 and older
- Why rates of HIV/AIDS are changing among this age group
- Some issues in treatment of older adults with HIV/AIDS

Although people are increasingly educated about HIV/AIDS, many stereotypes and misunderstandings still exist. One such idea is that older adults need not be concerned about HIV/AIDS. Data show, however, that the prevalence of HIV/AIDS is increasing among those aged 50 and older.[1] Yet neither older adults nor their physicians may recognize HIV/AIDS as a threat for this age group.

RATES OF HIV/AIDS AMONG OLDER ADULTS

People in the 50-plus age group accounted for roughly 10% of all new AIDS cases in the United States for most of the first two decades of the epidemic. In the late 1990s, however, this percentage began to increase. By 2005, people 50 years of age and older made up 19% of all AIDS diagnoses in the United States, 29% of those living with AIDS, and over one-third (35%) of all deaths due to AIDS (CDC, 2007).

Just as for younger age groups, HIV/AIDS cases among older adults vary by race and ethnic background with African Americans and Hispanics being

---

[1] Although much data addressing the health issues of older adults statistically includes only those aged 65 and older, the data on HIV/AIDS increasingly categorizes those aged 50 and above as "older adults."

overrepresented among older adults with HIV/AIDS (CDC, 2008). Older adults who are a member of a racial or ethnic minority may also experience longer delays in getting an accurate diagnosis of their condition or increased difficulties in seeking treatment (e.g., Zingmond et al., 2001).

WHY ARE RATES OF HIV/AIDS INCREASING AMONG THIS AGE GROUP?

As summarized by the National Institute on Aging (June 2004), several factors seem to be impacting this increase in HIV and AIDS among older adults. One factor is that advances in treatment are helping people with HIV/AIDS live longer, so there are more people living longer who actually contracted HIV when they were much younger. At this time, there is little data to suggest how long older people who are infected with HIV will live. It could be that medical advances help them to live the same average lifespan as those who are not HIV+.

A second factor in the increasing rates of HIV/AIDS among those aged 50 and older is that physicians are increasingly looking for, and thus, diagnosing HIV infection among this age group. In 2006, the CDC began to recommend routine HIV testing for all adults aged 18–64, not just those who had previously been considered in "high-risk" categories, such as intravenous drug users or men who have sex with men (CDC, 2006). HIV testing for those over age 64 is recommended only if there are known risk factors or symptoms suggestive of HIV/AIDS (Branson et al., 2006). Health care providers who follow these guidelines are now testing more older patients than in the past. However, all providers may still not actually test their older patients for HIV. The health care provider may feel testing is unnecessary. Also, like those of any other age group, older adults might be embarrassed or fearful of being tested. This lack of testing may actually mean that rate of HIV infection is even higher among older adults than the data show with unaware HIV+ individuals not taking precautions to avoid transmission.

Communication between health care providers and patients on the subject of HIV/AIDS can compound the problem. Health care professionals often do not talk with their older patients about drug use or safe sex practices (Lindau, 2007). Older patients themselves may, in turn, be reluctant to bring up such topics with their health care provider. These are concerns often seen, albeit incorrectly, as concerns involving only younger patients. For example, research shows that injection drug use (a high risk factor when needles are shared) has received little attention among older adults (Levy, 1998; Linsk, 2000).

Additionally, today's society is often accused of being youth-oriented and devaluing those who are aging, in particular stigmatizing those who are aging and ill. The stigma of HIV/AIDS as transmitted through drug abuse and sexual activity may be especially keen for older adults. The combination of these stigmas can be harsh as the statement made by a high-schooler to one older HIV+ activist reveals, "We're all going to die sometime. You're old. What's the big deal?" (HRSA Care Action, 2001).

Older adults also may know less about HIV/AIDS than younger people do. Often, they have never had any structured sex education programs like the ones that many schools offer, which teach about HIV/AIDS. They may also, for example, be dating after being widowed. Concern about HIV/AIDS was not part of dating as they previously experienced it, so it is not part of their current considerations either. Condom use, a safer sex practice that could curb the transmission of HIV, is infrequent among older adults no longer concerned with the need to prevent pregnancy (Williams and Donnelly, 2002). Older women, in particular, may be at risk of becoming infected when condoms are not used. This is due to vaginal tears that may occur during intercourse as a result of decreased lubrication and thinning of vaginal walls associated with normal aging (Catania et al., 1989). Drugs like Viagra and Cialis that increase sexual activity among the older population have been accused of compounding this problem. One positive result of the increasing rates of HIV/AIDS among older adults, and recognition of the factors discussed here, is that more attention is being directed toward educational efforts aimed at this age group.

TREATMENT CONCERNS SPECIFIC TO OLDER ADULTS WITH HIV/AIDS

There are few geriatric physicians who are experts in HIV/AIDS. When HIV/AIDS is discovered in an older person, it may be at a later stage, because the person has had the virus for quite some time, sometimes due to previous misdiagnoses. Or, they and their physician may have previously mistaken symptoms for "normal" aging before a proper diagnosis was made (Siegel, Dean, and Schrimshaw, 1999). The person may have been sick for some time but they were not tested for HIV because neither they nor their health care provider thought of it as a possibility.

Medical treatment for older adults with HIV/AIDS may involve specific challenges. For example, they may already be caregivers themselves of family or friends who are in need of care. Older adults may have fewer social supports in place to provide for their care than do younger individuals (Ory and Zablotsky, 1989). Immune system functions generally decline somewhat as aging progresses, so the opportunistic infections associated with HIV/AIDS may be more problematic among older persons.

Antiretroviral drug therapies that combat HIV may be particularly hard on older patients. These drug regimens may also interact with other medications taken by older individuals to combat a range of aging-related health problems. Older patients are not routinely included in drug trials, so the impact of pharmaceuticals on older bodies is not well-documented by solid research. Additionally, it may be difficult to determine whether symptoms such as dementia or slower mental processing are due to aging, HIV/AIDS, or drug therapy. Older people, however, may more strictly adhere to medication schedules than younger people do, and that is a particularly important factor in how well antiretroviral drugs are able to do their jobs.

REFERENCES

Branson, Bernard M., H. Hunter Handsfield, Margaret A. Lampe, Robert S. Janssen, Allan W. Taylor, Sheryl B. Lyss, and Jill E. Clark. September 22, 2006. "Revised Recommendations for HIV Testing of Adults, Adolescents, and Pregnant Women in Health-care Settings." *Morbidity and Mortality Weekly Report.* 55, RR-14:1–17. Accessed online May 2008. http://www.cdc.gov/mmwr/preview/mmwrhtml/rr5514a1.htm.

Catania, J.A., H. Turner, S.M. Kegeles, R. Stall, L. Pollack, and T.J. Coates. 1989. "Older Americans and AIDS: Transmission Risks and Primary Prevention Research Needs." *Gerontologist.* 29, 3: 373–381.

Centers for Disease Control and Prevention (CDC). 2007. *HIV/AIDS Surveillance Report, 2005.* Vol. 17. Rev. ed. Atlanta: U.S. Department of Health and Human Services, CDC: 1–54. Accessed online May 2008. http://www.cdc.gov/hiv/topics/surveillance/resources/reports/2005report/.

——. 2008. *HIV/AIDS Surveillance Report, 2006.* Vol. 18. Atlanta: U.S. Department of Health and Human Services, Centers for Disease Control and Prevention. Accessed online May 2008. http://www.cdc.gov/hiv/topics/surveillance/resources/reports/.

——. 2006. "Revised Recommendations for HIV Testing of Adults, Adolescents, and Pregnant Women in Health-Care Settings." *Morbidity and Mortality Weekly Report.* September 22, 2006 / 55(RR14): 1–17. Accessed online May 2008. http://www.cdc.gov/mmwr/preview/mmwrhtml/rr5514a1.htm.

HRSA Care Action. February 2001. "HIV Disease in Individuals Ages Fifty and Above." HIV/AIDS Bureau. Health Resources and Services Administration. Department of Health and Human Services. Rockville, MD: 3.

Levy, J. 1998. "AIDS and Injecting Drug Use in Later Life." *Research on Aging.* 20, 6: 1–13.

Lindau, S.T., M.A. Schumm, and E.O. Laumann EO, et al. 2007. "A Study of Sexuality and Health among Older Adults in the United States." *New England Journal of Medicine.* 357: 762–774.

Linsk, N.L. 2000. "HIV Among Older Adults." *AIDS Reader 2000*. 10, 7: 430–40.

National Institute on Aging. June 2004. "HIV, AIDS, and Older People." U.S. Department of Health and Human Services. Public Health Service. Washington, D.C.: National Institutes of Health. Accessed online May 2008. http://www.nia.nih.gov/HealthInformation/Publications/hiv-aids.htm.

Ory, M.G., and D. Zablotsky. 1989. "Notes for the Future: Research, Prevention, Care, Public Policy." In *AIDS in an Aging Society*. M.W. Riley, M.G. Ory, and D. Zablotsky, eds. New York, NY: Springer.

Siegel, K., L. Dean, and E. Schrimshaw. 1999. "Symptom Ambiguity among Late Middle-Aged and Older Adults with HIV." *Research on Aging*. 21, 4: 1–23.

Williams, E., and J. Donnelly. 2002. "Older Americans and AIDS: Some Guidelines for Prevention." *Social Work*. 47, 1: 1–7.

Zingmond, D.S., N.S. Wenger, S. Crystal, et al. 2001. "Circumstances at HIV Diagnosis and Progression of Disease in Older HIV-Infected Americans." *American Journal of Public Health*. 91: 1117–1120.

CHAPTER 13

Racial/Ethnic Inequality and HIV/AIDS

In this chapter, we will

- Demonstrate how race is not an accurate concept
- Discuss the harmful outcomes of categorizing people based on race or ethnicity
- Observe HIV/AIDS outcomes within different racial/ethnic groups

THE ILLUSION OF RACE

For better or worse (evidence from history seems to indicate the latter), humans have categorized people into different groups. Some categories are obvious due to clear physical and genetic differences, such as male and female. Others, such as race and ethnicity, are not. Recent scientific studies have indicated that despite the popular notion that there are distinct races of people, there is insufficient genetic evidence to support this claim. In other words, the notion of there being distinct races of people is a human construction, not a biological reality. This is not to say that there are not physical differences between different people whom we have traditionally characterized as being members of different races; clearly there are differences in skin tone, hair texture, facial features, and so on; no scientist denies this. Where the data are lacking is in terms of what these differences amount to.

Currently, the data indicate that the differences do not warrant placing humans into different racial categories (Wells, 2002). Similarly, mitochondrial DNA evidence continues to point to modern humans emerging from a common ancestor in what we now call the continent of Africa. Although there is some debate about this issue, most human evolutionary scientists conclude that humans arose in Africa and spread out from there in two migrations to populate the world. Taken together, the lack of genetic evidence to warrant separate racial categorizations and the mitochondrial DNA evidence that humans have a common ancestor, these two sources of data provide evidence that the notion of there being distinct races of people is inaccurate. As noted, however, the categorization of peoples into different races persists.

DISCRIMINATION

Categorization of peoples in and of itself is not necessarily bad; what makes this process harmful is the unequal distribution of valuable social resources that accompanies it. In other words, historically, people have been entitled to receive more socially valuable resources (money, prestige, opportunity) simply because of the categories they have been placed into at birth. Evidence of this in the United States in particular is easily found. Women were not considered capable of participating in political activities until the early 1900s, as it was believed that politics was a "masculine" pursuit; as such, we see an unequal representation of women in political positions in the United States, that is, there are more men than women in positions of political power even though the number of men and women in the United States is roughly the same. The United States has limited other groups from full participation in certain social activities; African Americans have been singularly targeted for discrimination throughout history—for example, by "Jim Crow" laws, by prohibition of home ownership, and by being used as unsuspecting guinea pigs in research on the progression of syphilis.

Fortunately, there have been remedies to most of these harmful practices through the enactment of legislation, extensive public education, and increased public awareness of discrimination as common practice. One seemingly innocent endeavor has been to recategorize people into different ethnic groups as a way to respect differences between people. This has not proven to be that successful, however, because for many, ethnic identification has simply replaced racial identification. In other words, instead of referring to someone as Black, she or he is now referred to as African American. In practice, this recategorization has not resulted in less discrimination necessarily, it has simply resulted in a new name for an old category.

Similarly, the notion of distinct ethnic categories does not necessarily stand up to scientific scrutiny, because there are many overlapping "ethnic" elements among and between groups. One example will demonstrate the problems with this notion of differing "ethnic groups." Consider African Americans again. Does a "White" person born in Zimbabwe (a country in Africa) who becomes a naturalized American citizen refer to her- or himself as "African American"? Or how is a "Black" person born and raised in the United States inherently familiar with the "ethnic" practices of any groups of people in Africa? Modern African Americans, whose ancestors were brought to the United States as slaves and were not afforded an opportunity to maintain a connection of any kind to their ancestral homeland, are largely unsure of where and with what group in Africa they can claim a cultural heritage (there are thousands of tribes within the continent of Africa). So, inasmuch as there have been attempts (presumably in the spirit of fairness and reconciliation) to ameliorate the effects of past discriminatory practices, some have been more successful than others.

Despite efforts at reducing or eliminating harmful practices, there are, however, unfortunate lingering effects from generations of discrimination for certain groups of people. The one effect that concerns us here is the differential HIV/AIDS outcomes for people based on their race or ethnicity.

Below, we will examine prevalence rates and other HIV/AIDS data in the United States as these are divided into racial/ethnic categories; international data are generally not divided this way, as they tend to be aggregated by country and then by other sociodemographics such as gender, education level, poverty level, and so forth. As noted above, these reveal a continuing pattern of an unequal distribution of resources. We will focus on two racial/ethnic groups that historically have been victims of intentional discrimination and demonstrate empirically the impact of the lasting effects of the categorization of people.

AFRICAN AMERICANS

In 2005, the CDC reported that despite the fact that African Americans comprised 13% of the total population in the 2000 U.S. Census, they alone accounted for an estimated 37% of new HIV/AIDS cases in the United States (CDC, 2008b). In addition, the rate for AIDS diagnosis was 10 times higher among African Americans than among Anglophone whites and three times higher than among Hispanics. More specifically, the rate of AIDS diagnosis was 23 times higher for African American women than Anglophone white women and eight times higher for African American men than Anglophone white men. Transmission routes for African American men were highest among men having sex with other men; IDU transmission was second, and high-risk heterosexual contact third. African American women were most likely to become HIV+ through high-risk heterosexual sex followed by IDU. In that same year, 65% of infants perinatally infected with HIV were African American. Unfortunately, African Americans being at higher risk for HIV infection and AIDS is not new. The data indicate that they have accounted for 42% of all AIDS cases in the United States since the epidemic began.

The CDC indicates that there are several reasons that may account for the differences between African Americans and Anglophone whites. Some of these include lower likelihood of awareness of HIV status, higher rates of sexually-transmitted diseases in general, lower likelihood of acknowledging homosexual behavior, and higher likelihood of living in poverty (CDC, 2008b). This latter likelihood is related to higher incidence of HIV infection across virtually all groups. Data from other sources also indicate that people living in poverty have less chance of access to quality medical care, are less likely to seek medical care, and have fewer financial and other resources to adequately provide for basic human needs.

HISPANIC AMERICANS

The CDC reports that in 2005, the fourth leading cause of death for individuals between the ages of 35 to 44 was HIV/AIDS (CDC, 2008a). Similar to African Americans, there was a disproportionate number of Hispanic Americans reporting new HIV infections in 2005; comprising 15% of the total population of the United States, they accounted for 17% of known new infections. In 2006, Hispanic Americans represented 17% of all persons living with AIDS, 19% of new AIDS infections, and 19% of children living with HIV/AIDS.

Routes of transmission for Hispanic American males in 2006 included (in order of prevalence) men having sex with other men, IDU, and high-risk heterosexual behavior. For Hispanic American women, routes of transmission (again in order of prevalence) were high-risk heterosexual sex and IDU.

In accounting for these differences, the CDC reports that some of the factors include an inhibition among women to discuss the use of condoms, inconsistent use of condoms by men having sex with other men, substance abuse, higher rates than Anglos of sexually transmitted diseases, traditional gender roles that result in differences of power between men and women, and socioeconomic challenges (22% of Hispanic Americans live in poverty). Results of this latter factor include insufficient formal education, lack of awareness about HIV/AIDS, lowered access to quality medical care, lower likelihood of having insurance, and persistent un- and/or underemployment.

SUMMARY

The data presented above demonstrate that there are different health outcomes for people simply based on socially constructed categories. As noted, the concepts of race and ethnicity really don't stand up to thorough empirical analysis. Despite this, they persist among the general public and are firmly believed to be properties of human biology and are, as such, unchangeable. Categorization of people is not inherently harmful; what makes it harmful is when socially valuable resources such as wealth, income, access to health care, education, opportunity, and other resources, are distributed differently based on categorical membership. Because of these mistaken beliefs (e.g., African Americans are not as intelligent as other groups, Hispanic Americans are all in the country illegally), a disproportionate number of people in the discriminated categories experience more suffering and harm due to HIV/AIDS than individuals in other categories.

REFERENCES

Centers for Disease Control and Prevention (CDC). 2008a. "Hispanics/Latinos." CDC Web Site. Accessed online December 2008. http://www.cdc.gov/hiv/hispanics/index.htm.

_____. 2008b. "HIV/AIDS and African Americans." CDC Web Site. Accessed online December 2008. http://www.cdc.gov/hiv/topics/aa/index.htm.

Wells, Spencer. 2002. *The Journey of Man: A Genetic Odyssey*. New York: Random House Trade Paperback.

CHAPTER 14

The Gay, Lesbian, Bisexual, and Transgender (GLBT) Community and HIV/AIDS

In this chapter, we will

- Examine the prevalence of HIV/AIDS among men who have sex with men
- Discuss transmission among women who have sex with women
- Identify HIV/AIDS issues specific to the transgender community

MEN WHO HAVE SEX WITH MEN (MSM)

Because HIV is sexually transmitted, sexual behavior is a critical factor in the pandemic and has been afforded much attention. Particular attention has been directed toward men who have sex with men (MSM). The term "MSM" is generally used in discussing HIV/AIDS data rather than the label "homosexual." That is because sexual behavior and orientation defy simple categorizations or labeling. Some men who have sex with men will identify themselves as gay; some will identify themselves as bisexual; some will identify themselves as straight. The term MSM bypasses these labels and gets directly at activities that have the potential to transmit HIV. Men having sex with men frequently involves activities such as anal intercourse that, during unprotected sex, have a greater likelihood of transmitting HIV than does penile-vaginal intercourse (Engel, 2006; Kingsley, 1990; Pembrey, 2008). (The sidebar on "Bug-Chasers and

Gift-Givers" discusses a controversial mode of HIV transmission among a small MSM subculture.) Additionally, as concerns about HIV transmission from bisexual men to heterosexual women have grown, increasing attention has been placed on men on the "down low." "Down low" is a slang term that is

> often used to describe the behavior of men who have sex with other men as well as women and who do not identify as gay or bisexual. These men may refer to themselves as being "on the down low," "on the DL," or "on the low low." The term has most often been associated with African American men. Although the term originated in the African American community, the behaviors associated with the term are not new and not specific to black men who have sex with men. (CDC, 2006b)

In the United States, the earliest cases of the disease that would come to be known as AIDS were reported in self-identified gay men in San Francisco, California, and New York City, New York. The number of cases quickly grew among members of these gay communities, leading to early associations of HIV and AIDS with gay men and inaccurate and stigmatizing terms for AIDS such as the "gay plague" or "gay cancer." While these names for AIDS have fallen out of widespread usage, the assumption that men who contract HIV are gay or have engaged in sex with other men still colors responses to HIV/AIDS. Coupled with widespread homophobic attitudes, the legacy has been a long history of hateful stigma and discrimination targeting gays. (See Chapter 5 for a more in-depth discussion of the impact of this history.)

According to CDC data, rates of HIV/AIDS remain high among MSM. At the end of 2006, over 199,000 men in the United States were living with AIDS as a result of male-to-male transmission. Another 27,500 men with AIDS had engaged in both MSM and injection drug use. Together, these categories account for around 52% of people living with AIDS in the country, and 56% of AIDS deaths in the United States (2008b).

In 2006, 53% of all new HIV infections occurring that year (in both males and females) in the United States were in MSM. In looking only at new infection among men, 72% of all such infections were in MSM. This represents 81% of new infections among whites, 63% among blacks, and 72% among Hispanics. Higher percentages of new HIV infections among black and Hispanic men than among white men are from intravenous drug use and high-risk heterosexual activities. Yet the data on MSM transmission still show disproportionate numbers of blacks and Hispanics becoming infected. In the 13–29 age group, the number of new HIV infections in blacks (5,220, or 48%) was 1.6 times the number in whites (3,330, or

BUG-CHASERS AND GIFT-GIVERS

Not everyone wants to avoid contracting or transmitting HIV. A small and largely underground subculture of gay men, facilitated primarily by the Internet, consists of "bug-chasers," those seeking to become infected with HIV, and "gift-givers," those who are willing to give HIV to others. Bug-chasers and gift-givers may meet one-on-one or at seroconversion parties, in which a number of HIV− and HIV+ men have bareback sex (without using a condom). The HIV− participants may contract HIV, converting to HIV+ status (hence the term "seroconversion").

The reasons behind bug-chasing and gift-giving are complex and not well-researched. HIV may variously be seen as a sexy and erotic thrill, a symbol of connection in the gay community, a way to gain attention, a reflection of the incorrect assumption that advances in HIV medications have made HIV just another chronic illness and "no big deal," lack of self-esteem, or even a form of suicide to deal with issues such as heterosexism and discrimination. For some bug-chasers, intentionally contracting HIV is apparently hastening what they see as inevitable, eventually contracting the virus anyway, or blamed on having tired of the need to practice "safer-sex" to remain uninfected.

Bug-chasing and gift-giving are extremely controversial practices. They are widely scorned in the gay community and among AIDS advocacy groups. No reliable estimates exist on how many bug-chasers and gift-givers there are, but the numbers appear to be small.

REFERENCES

Freeman, Gregory A. 2003. "Bug Chasers: The Men Who Long to be HIV+." January 23. *Rolling Stone*. Accessed November 2008. http://www.rollingstone.com/news/story/5933610/bug_chasers.

Gauthier, D. K., and C. J. Forsyth. 1999. "Bareback Sex, Bug Chasing, and the Gift of Death." *Deviant Behavior*. 20, 1: 85−100.

"The Gift." 2003. Louise Hogarth, Director. Dream Out Loud Films.

Grov, C., and J.T. Parsons. 2006. "Bugchasing and Giftgiving: The Potential for HIV Transmission among Barebackers on the Internet." *AIDS Education and Prevention*. 18, 6: 490−503.

Tewksbury, R. 2006. "'Click Here for HIV': An Analysis of Internet-Based Bug Chasers and Bug Givers." *Deviant Behavior*. 27, 4: 379−395.

31%) and 2.3 times the number in Hispanics (2,300, or 21%) (CDC, 2008b).

WOMEN WHO HAVE SEX WITH WOMEN (WSW)

Women who have sex with women (WSW) who self-identify as lesbian or bisexual are generally not considered at high risk for contracting HIV through female-to-female sexual contact. Relatively few cases of female-to-female HIV transmission have been documented. Reports from the CDC do not even identify a category for female-to-female transmission. However, information on whether HIV+ women had sex with women is missing in much of the CDC data on this population, so there is some question as to whether the rates of female-to-female transmission are actually higher than known (CDC, 2006a).

What is clear is that women having sex with women involves risks that women should be aware of so they can properly protect themselves and their partners. Some women (possibly a high percentage) who engage in same-sex relationships have had sex with men. Some women use intravenous drugs, share needles for tattooing or piercing, or engage in other high-risk behaviors (e.g., Scheer et al, 2002). One confirmed case of female-to-female HIV transmission involved a female couple in which one partner identified as bisexual. Transmission occurred through activities involving sex toys and oral sex (Kwakwa et al., 2003). WSW are increasingly being encouraged to engage in HIV prevention practices and get tested for HIV.

TRANSGENDER AND HIV/AIDS

An often overlooked subset of individuals with HIV infection are those in the transgender community. The term "transgender" involves complex and evolving concepts. It incorporates *transsexuals* (those who medically alter the biological sex they are born with, or choose to live as a member of the other sex without medical alteration), as well as *intersexuals* (those born with indeterminate sex characteristics or with those of both male and female), and *transvestites* (people who dress as members of the opposite sex) (Benokraitis, 2008). Some transgender people identify themselves as either male or female. Others identify themselves through the use of two gender identity categories. "Male-to-females (MTFs) are people whose birth-assigned gender is male, but whose gender identity is female, and female-to-males (FTMs) are people whose birth-assigned gender is female, but whose gender identity is male" (Kenagy, 2008).[1] Although no one knows for sure an exact number of transgender individuals living in the United States, perhaps 2% of Americans are transgender (Gorman, 1995).

The rate of HIV in the transgender community is hard to estimate. This data has not been systematically tracked on a nationwide level, so the numbers that we do have come from smaller scale research conducted in various locations around the country. Some research estimates the rate of HIV among transgender people to be something less than 12%. Other research finds rates to be higher, sometimes much higher, ranging to 69% (Berry, 2008; CDC, n.d.; Herbst, 2008). The transgender rates of HIV infection are highest among minorities, sex workers, and MTF transgender individuals as compared to FTMs.

Transgender individuals who are HIV+ are faced with some unique challenges not shared by others with HIV. Social stigma and discrimination against transgender people and their partners can be obstacles in their efforts to develop long-term relationships and potentially exclusive sexual partners. Stigmas and discrimination may also be factors in transgender individuals sometimes feeling socially isolated or having low self-esteem, both of which may lead to some engaging in sexual activity for social connections or person affirmation. Other problems for the transgender community that may increase rates of HIV transmission or lead to additional problems for those who are already HIV+ include engaging in sex work, not following safer sex practices, using intravenous drugs and sharing needles, being subjected to physical and other forms of abuse, having unmet transgender-specific health care needs, and the many unmet educational and prevention needs among the transgendered community itself as well as policymakers and service providers (Berry, 2008; Bockting and Avery, 2006; CDC, n.d.; Herbst et al., 2008; Jones, 2008; Kenagy, 2008).

For HIV+ transgendered people, hormone therapies intended to make individuals physically more masculine or more feminine mean some specific challenges to their HIV treatment regimes. These hormone therapies are lifelong therapies. They have not been laboratory tested for drug

---

[1] We use the terms "sex," "gender," "gender identity," and "sexual orientation" often in everyday conversation. However, sometimes they are improperly used as if they are interchangeable terms. These terms actually have specific definitions that are important to understanding the term "transgender." Sex is the biological characteristics at birth which determine whether a person is male or female. *Gender* is the attitudes and behaviors that society considers masculine or feminine, and that characterize males and females respectively. *Gender identity* is a person's awareness that they are male or female, or as the term implies, the gender with which they identify themselves. *Sexual orientation* is a person's sexual attraction to the opposite or same sex, or both sexes.

interactions and may interact with HIV medications (Vazquez, 2008a, 2008b). They may also sometimes involve risky needle sharing.

Resources for, and attention to, the transgender community is increasing. An Internet search on transgender and HIV will lead to many resources ranging from health care information, to social support, to advocacy, and more. Several readable articles and an annotated listing of Web addresses for further information are available in the July/August 2008 "Transgender and HIV" edition of *Positively Aware,* the journal of the Test Positive Aware Network. The Network also provides an online collection of links to a wide range of information on HIV infection and transgender issues at http://positivelyaware.com/2008/08_04/resources.html.

REFERENCES

Benokraitis, Nijole V. 2008. *Marriages and Families: Changes, Choices, and Constraints,* 6th ed. Upper Saddle River, NJ: Pearson/Prentice Hall.

Berry, Jeff. 2008. "An Interview with Walter Bockting, Ph.D." *Positively Aware.* 19, 4: 38–39.

Bockting, Walter, and Eric Avery. 2006. *Transgender Health and HIV Prevention: Needs Assessment Studies from Transgender Communities Across the United States.* Binghamton, NY: Haworth Medical Press.

Centers for Disease Control and Prevention (CDC). 2008a. *HIV/AIDS Surveillance Report, 2006.* 18. Atlanta: U.S. Department of Health and Human Services, CDC Web site. Accessed online November 2008. http://www.cdc.gov/hiv/topics/surveillance/resources/reports/.

———. No date. "HIV/AIDS and Transgender Persons." CDC Web site. Accessed online September 2008. http://www.cdc.gov/lgbthealth/pdf/FS-Transgender-06192007.pdf.

———. 2006a. "HIV/AIDS among Women Who Have Sex With Women." CDC Web site. Accessed online December 2008. http://www.cdc.gov/hiv/topics/women/resources/factsheets/wsw.htm.

———. 2006b. "Questions and Answers: Men on the Down Low." CDC Web site. Accessed online December 2008. http://www.cdc.gov/hiv/topics/aa/resources/qa/downlow.htm.

———. 2008b. "Subpopulation Estimates from the HIV Incidence Surveillance System— United States, 2006." *Morbidity and Mortality Weekly Report.* September 12. 57, 36: 985–989. CDC Web site. Accessed online December 2008. http://www.cdc.gov/hiv/topics/msm/resources/factsheets/msm.htm.

Engel, Jonathan. 2006. *The Epidemic: A Global History of AIDS.* New York: Smithsonian.

Gorman, C. 1995. "Trapped in the Body of a Man?" *Time.* Nov 13: 94–95.

Herbst, Jeffrey H., Elizabeth D. Jacobs, Teresa J. Finlayson, Vel S. McKleroy, Mary Spink Neumann, and Nicole Crepaz. 2008. "Estimating HIV Prevalence and Risk Behaviors of Transgender Persons in the United States: A Systematic Review." *AIDS and Behavior*. 12, 1: 1–17.

Jones, Laura. 2008. "Safer Sex Post-SRS: A Brave New World, Indeed." *Positively Aware*. 19, 4: 51–54.

Kenagy, Gretchen P. 2008. "The Invisible." *Positively Aware*. 19, 4: 18–19.

Kingsley, L.A., C.R. Rinaldo Jr., D.W. Lyter, R.O. Valdiserri, S.H. Belle, and M. Ho. 1990. "Sexual Transmission Efficiency of Hepatitis B Virus and Human Immunodeficiency Virus among Homosexual Men." *JAMA*. 264, 2: 230–234.

Kwakwa, Helena A., and M.W. Ghobrial. 2003. "Female-to-Female Transmission of Human Immunodeficiency Virus." *Clinical Infectious Diseases*. 36, 3: e40–e41.

Pembrey, Graham. 2008. "HIV, AIDS, and Men Who Have Sex with Men." November 12. AVERTing HIV and AIDS (AVERT) Web site. Accessed December 2008. http://www.avert.org/msm.htm.

Scheer, Susan, Ingrid Peterson, Kimberly Page-Shafer, Viva Delgado, Alice Gleghorn, Juan Ruiz, Fred Molitor, William McFarland, Jeffrey Klausner, and the Young Women's Survey Team. 2002. "Sexual and Drug Use Behavior Among Women Who Have Sex With Both Women and Men: Results of a Population-Based Survey." *American Journal of Public Health*. 92, 7: 1110–1112.

Vazquez, Enid. 2008a. "Transgender Therapy and HIV." *Positively Aware*. 19, 4: 20–22.

_____. 2008b. "A Transgender Therapy Primer." *Positively Aware*. 19, 4: 46–48.

CHAPTER 15

Drug Users and HIV/AIDS

In this chapter, we will discuss

- The prevalence of substance abuse in the United States and internationally
- The relationship between substance abuse and transmission of HIV
- The prevalence of substance users that are HIV-positive
- Prevention efforts regarding HIV transmission among drug users

PREVALENCE OF SUBSTANCE ABUSE

Substance abuse is not a new phenomenon. Psychoactive substances have been used by human beings for millennia (Rudgley, 1993). There is evidence that people used opium as far back as 6,000 years ago (Ksir, Ray and Oakley, 2006). Indeed, psychoactive substances have been part of the human condition since prehistory and are a part of the human condition today. Many people associate substance use with the use of illegal drugs such as marijuana, heroin, and ecstasy to alter or enhance one's experience. In fact, more people use legal substances to do this and do so on a daily basis; consider the number of people that use nicotine, caffeine, and alcohol around the world. When one stops to consider the amount of substance used by human beings on a daily basis to alter the way that they feel, how much energy they have, or decrease anxiety, the number is overwhelming.

It is really no surprise that the numbers are so high. All of these substances work on a neurological level; they all modify or change the way that nerve cells (specifically neurons) interact with one another. It is well documented that changing the way that neurons communicate by manipulating the means of transmission (neurotransmitters) results in those very things that people seek when they use substances—effects such as increased energy, decreased anxiety, and increased excitement.

Substance use becomes problematic when it begins to interfere with one's ability to successfully carry out life's responsibilities; it is at this point that it is defined as either abuse or dependence. The sidebar to this chapter defines both of these concepts. It is typically those people who abuse substances who are at a much higher risk for HIV infection and subsequent transmission.

DEFINING SUBSTANCE ABUSE AND SUBSTANCE DEPENDENCE

In its *Diagnostic and Statistical Manual of Mental Disorders,* the American Psychiatric Association distinguishes between *substance abuse* and *substance dependence*. The criteria for diagnosing substance abuse are:

> A pattern of substance use leading to significant impairment in functioning. One of the following must be present within a 12-month period: (1) recurrent use resulting in a failure to fulfill major obligations at work, school, or home; (2) recurrent use in situations which are physically hazardous (e.g., driving while intoxicated); (3) legal problems resulting from recurrent use; or (4) continued use despite significant social or interpersonal problems caused by the substance use. The symptoms do not meet the criteria for substance dependence as abuse is a part of this disorder.

The criteria for diagnosing substance dependence are:

> Substance use history which includes the following: (1) substance abuse (see above); (2) continuation of use despite related problems; (3) increase in tolerance (more of the drug is needed to achieve the same effect); and (4) withdrawal symptoms.

REFERENCE

American Psychiatric Association (APA). 2000. *Diagnostic and Statistical Manual of Mental Disorders (DSM-IV-TR),* Fourth Edition. Arlington, VA: American Psychiatric Publishing.

The Substance Abuse and Mental Health Services Administration (SAMHSA, 2007) is a federal agency that, among its many functions, collects an annual survey ("The National Survey on Drug Use and Health") on substance use by Americans aged 12 and older. There are nine different categories of drugs that respondents are reported on marijuana, cocaine, heroin, hallucinogens, inhalants, and the nonmedical use of prescription-type pain relievers, tranquilizers, stimulants, and sedatives (SAMHSA, 2007). The most recent data from 2007 reveal that there were almost 20 million Americans aged 12 and older who had used an illicit drug in the month prior to the survey (SAMHSA, 2007). This represents 8% of the population and is a slight decrease from the 8.3% of people that reported using an illicit substance in 2006. Marijuana was the drug most frequently reported (14.4 million people), followed by psychotherapeutics (6.9 million), cocaine (2.1 million), hallucinogens (1.0 million), inhalants (0.6 million), and heroin (0.2 million) (SAMHSA, 2007). The reported use of these substances has remained fairly stable over the last five years, with only minimal changes in percent of persons using (SAMHSA, 2007).

The WHO also collects data on substance abuse, but on a global scale. The most recent data on the use of specific substances were collected from 1998 to 2001 and indicated that there were 185 million people using substances worldwide. 69% (148 million people) used marijuana, 16% (33.4 million) used amphetamines, 6% (13.4 million) used cocaine, 6% (12.9 million) used heroin or other opiates, and 3% (7 million) used MDMA (Ecstasy) (WHO, 2008b).Though they define problematic substance use differently than SAMHSA, their data are still compelling. Their current estimates are that 15.3 million persons worldwide have drug use disorders (WHO, 2008a). Intravenous drug use (IDU) is reported in 136 countries, and of those, 93 report HIV infection among the IDU population (WHO, 2008a).

RELATIONSHIP BETWEEN SUBSTANCE ABUSE AND TRANSMISSION OF HIV

As has been discussed in this text already, transmission of HIV occurs when there is an opportunity for the virus to remain viable during transfer from one person to another. The "best" opportunity for spread of infection between one person and another is through the immediate transfer of infected bodily fluids. As is also well known, many persons use substances intravenously. One of the reasons that they use this particular method of administration is that the substance enters directly into the bloodstream and gets to the brain very rapidly. In other words, one can get "high" faster and with a bigger impact if one uses the intravenous method of substance administration. This, in and of itself is not problematic when it comes to the transmission of HIV (although, as we will see, by simply using substances, one puts oneself at risk for engaging in risky behavior), because simply injecting substances does not transmit HIV infection. The problem enters when those that are using intravenously (IDU) begin to share syringes with each other. Many IDUs will first draw blood into the syringe and then depress the plunger, injecting the substance into the vein. Inevitably, not all of their blood is injected back into the vein, so if they pass the syringe along to others to use, they also pass along small portions of their blood. Similarly, one might not inject the entire amount directly into his or her vein, but inject a portion and then share the remainder in the syringe with others. In all of these cases, there is a very high risk of transmitting HIV with a contaminated syringe.

Of course, another way to spread HIV is through sexual contact; this too is related to the abuse of substances (NIDA, 2006). As noted, substances have an impact on a neurological level. One result is that people who abuse substances tend to make different choices while intoxicated. This is because their brain is literally different when under the influence. The neurological connections do not work in the same way when the person is using substances. This results in global changes in the ability to assess situations, determine risk, think logically, and ultimately make good decisions. Of course, these failures in judgment apply to whatever it is they are doing while intoxicated, including deciding to have sex and with whom. Unfortunately, this often results in individuals engaging in unsafe sexual practices, which significantly increases the risk of HIV transmission.

It is also not unusual for substance users to trade sex for drugs. In these cases, the person might not be under the influence before or after engaging in sex, but may be less concerned with ensuring that safe sexual practices are observed because of the pressing need to obtain the substance. One consequence of physical dependence is physical withdrawal symptoms when the level of the substance in the blood stream decreases. This results in painful sensations and cravings for the dependent person. As such, the physical need for the substance is overpowering, so much so, that securing the substance through any means becomes the immediate goal. As noted, this results in many people not practicing safe sex and thereby increasing the risk of transmission.

Finally, use of substances can have a deteriorating impact on the body. In some cases, this is due to the substance itself; in other cases, this is due to the lack of self care often associated with substance abuse. Deteriorating health, for whatever reason, increases the chances of successful HIV transmission. Recall that HIV attacks cells within the immune system; having an already weakened immune system due to drug use and associated factors can accelerate HIV infection and also the development of AIDS. It is not that substance abusers don't care about their health; rather it is the draw of the substance, both psychologically and physically, that makes securing and using the substance a primary goal in life. Many substance abusers are incapable of holding jobs, maintaining caring relationships with others, or managing money, among other tasks. These behavioral deficits, which are intimately related to their substance abuse, result in an inability to adequately care for themselves, thus making them more prone to infection. Similarly, when a substance abuser is HIV positive, continued use of substances generally hastens the diagnosis of AIDS and can increase the likelihood of secondary infection by an opportunistic illness.

PREVALENCE OF SUBSTANCE USERS THAT ARE HIV POSITIVE

Despite the knowledge that substance abuse in general can lead to increased likelihood of HIV infection, most of the data collected on substance abuse and HIV status come from IDUs. This is perhaps due to the fact that IDUs can directly transmit the virus to other IDUs. Also, intravenous drug use was one of the first recognized means of transmission. All health professionals acknowledge that substance abuse of any kind can lead to a greatly increased risk of HIV transmission, however.

The most recent report from the WHO on IDUs and HIV status estimates that there are approximately 15 million IDUs (less than 1% of the world's population) internationally, and of those, approximately, 3 to 4 million (20% to 27%) are HIV positive (WHO, 2008c). In 2000, the CDC reported that IDU accounted for 36% of all reported AIDS cases, and of all of the new AIDS cases reported in 2000 alone, 28% were associated with IDU. Data from the most recent CDC surveillance study estimated that 14% of HIV-infected Americans received it through intravenous drug transmission (CDC, 2006). Of course, it is not just IDUs who are at risk of becoming infected; it is also those people who are in relationships with IDUs. CDC data from 2000 indicated that 13% of sex partners, 13% of men having sex with male IDUs, and 1% of children of IDUs or their sex partner had been diagnosed with AIDS (CDC, 2002).

As these data indicate, IDUs and HIV transmission are closely related. As such, prevention and treatment efforts for both conditions need to be coordinated. Unfortunately, dependency on substances compounds the problem of prevention and treatment of both conditions. The current understanding of substance abuse and dependency is much improved since these conditions became social issues, but it is as yet incomplete. What is known permits effective intervention; however, it is also well known that successful treatment of both substance abuse and dependence is difficult. This is in part due to the nature of abuse and dependency; both result in unhealthy lifestyles and impaired decision-making. As noted previously, impaired decision-making due to substance abuse or dependence puts one at increased risk of HIV infection, but it also results in individuals not following through with prevention and intervention efforts to treat abuse or dependence. In other words, many substance abusers are unable to see the need to moderate or abstain from the use of substances and often continue using despite serious personal consequences. Substance dependence in particular is difficult to treat because the dependence is physical. Refraining from using a substance that one is dependent upon is similar to being extremely dehydrated or famished; both conditions are physically painful. When one is in the state of withdrawal, the simple use of the substance beings immediate relief; this is a difficult dynamic to contend with when a health professional is attempting to encourage the dependent user that abstinence is the best option.

PREVENTION EFFORTS

As is obvious from reading the previous sections of this chapter, a number of behaviors need to be addressed when it comes to preventing HIV transmission among this population. In many ways, this is the probably the most difficult population to treat. Space limitations prevent us from delving into all of the possible options, so we will focus on two in particular; preventing the use of substances in general and decreasing the likelihood of transmission among IDUs.

Within the last thirty years, billions of dollars have been spent on the prevention of the use of substances. As a result, the overall use of substances has declined; however, it still remains a problem throughout the world. One reason is that the production, distribution and sales of illicit substances is very profitable. The other is that substances have a profound impact on an individual, both psychologically and physically; both responses very often increase the motivation for continued use.

Currently, most prevention efforts focus on reducing the flow of illicit substances into a population (mainly through law enforcement) and through education on the effects and dangers of using substances. Taken together, these have resulted in decreases as noted above. Another approach that is gaining ground, but requires much more structural change, hence its lack of widespread presence, is "insulating" adolescents against risky behaviors by carefully monitoring their primary socialization. The overall idea is to provide them with opportunities and support to develop good decision-making skills, affirm pro-social values, learn to think critically, and find reward in being helpful and productive. The best example of this approach is the work done by the Search Institute, which after years of research has identified 40 developmental assets that dramatically decrease the likelihood of drug use and other risky behaviors (SEARCH, 2008).

The objective to all of these approaches is to prevent adolescents (or anyone else) from even starting to use substances. Those that do not use any substances are therefore not at risk for contributing to those behaviors that are detrimental to society, which in this context are behaviors that would give rise to an increased likelihood of HIV transmission or the hastening of the development of AIDS. Since prevention is the primary goal, one would expect that there would be data on the efficacy of different prevention approaches. Unfortunately, prevention is virtually impossible to measure. The reason for this is that researchers never know the number of people who might engage in a behavior without prevention efforts; in other words, the knowledge that we have about human behavior is not complete enough to allow anyone to determine who might need prevention efforts and who might not.

When the above-mentioned primary prevention efforts fail and individuals abuse or become dependent on substances, other approaches can be employed. Again, due to space limitations, we will focus on those efforts that have been developed in response to IDUs. These approaches are recommended throughout the world.

As we have been discussing, IDUs are at a very high risk for both HIV infection and acceleration to AIDS once infected due to the use of substances and their means of administration (syringes). Knowing this has resulted in several different approaches that can decrease the likelihood of HIV transmission. Two ubiquitous methods that will not be discussed are HIV/AIDS education and substance abuse treatment programs. Both of these interventions vary in terms of success, quality, and availability, however, both approaches are employed to reduce the transmission of HIV.

One of the first approaches developed was the syringe exchange program (CDC, 2005). Since many IDUs share syringes and other paraphernalia, providing them with clean needles was thought to reduce the risk of spreading HIV. (See Figure 15.1.) This has worked with varying levels of success. Many health professionals recommend this strategy because, if nothing else, it does result in a decreased number of infected items available to users. In addition, when IDUs exchange syringes at a medical facility, they have the opportunity to discuss HIV/AIDS, IDU, treatment options, and counseling with health professionals. This latter function of the exchange program can oftentimes be the most valuable aspect, because it provides the IDU with a known and trusted contact if and when he or she decides to make healthier life choices, such as abstaining from use or seeking medical care.

Another approach that targets the use of syringes is educating IDUs about how to use bleach and other cleaning agents to disinfect their syringes and other IV paraphernalia. Exchange of syringes is a better option, but when those services are unavailable, thorough disinfecting is better than not doing anything. Of course, not sharing syringes is the best

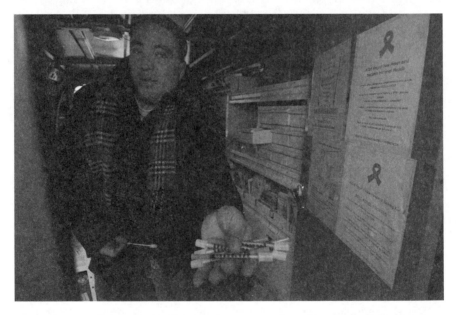

Figure 15.1 George Ducheli, who drives a van for a New Haven, Connecticut, needle exchange program, displays syringes while posing for a photograph in the program's van before going out to exchange needles and syringes from addicts. A growing body of research has found that needle exchange programs reduce the spread of AIDS without increasing drug use. However, local budget cuts and a federal ban on funding such programs in the U.S. and abroad are hurting the programs at a time when injection drug use is fueling a global AIDS epidemic, advocates say. (Courtesy AP Photo/Douglas Healey.)

option (if such a thing as a "best" option is possible when using IV), but many IDUs lack the resources or decision-making to observe this practice.

In the prevalence section above, we noted that individuals in relationships with IDUs were also at a high risk for becoming infected. Aside from the potential of transmission due to the sharing of IV paraphernalia, most significant others of IDUs are put at risk through unsafe sexual practices. As such, another prevention effort, the distribution of condoms and accompanying education on their use and limitations, is recommended by many health professionals. Using condoms does not guarantee lack of possibility of transmission, but it does decrease the risk for both the IDU and those with whom she or he is in a relationship with.

SUMMARY

Substance abuse is an ongoing social problem with a long, historical precedent. The likelihood of human beings never using substances is very remote. Substance abuse and HIV/AIDS have been linked from the very beginning of the recognition of the virus and accompanying syndrome. Substance abusers are one of the more difficult populations to treat due to the nature of how substances affect the brain and also due to the general social condemnation of illicit substance use. Due to the severity of HIV/AIDS, however, health professionals have developed both prevention and treatment options that, if employed effectively, can reduce the likelihood of continued HIV transmission. The extent to which any or all of the developed options are utilized depends on many factors determined in large part by the communities of which IDUs are members. It is quite obvious from the data that continued prevention and treatment efforts are very much in demand.

REFERENCES

Centers for Disease Control and Prevention (CDC). 2002. *Drug-associated HIV Transmission Continues in the United States.* CDC Web site. Accessed online November 2008. http://www.cdc.gov/hiv/resources/factsheets/idu.htm.

_____. 2005. *Syringe Exchange Programs.* CDC Web site. Accessed online November 2008. http://www.cdc.gov/idu/facts/AED_IDU_SYR.pdf.

_____. 2006. *Table 18. Reported Cases of HIV Infection (Not AIDS) by Age Category, Transmission Category, and Sex, 2006 and Cumulative—45 States and 5 U.S. Dependent Areas with Confidential Name-Based HIV Infection Reporting.* CDC Web site. Accessed online November 2008. http://www.cdc.gov/hiv/topics/surveillance/resources/reports/2006report/table18.htm.

Ksir, C.J., Hart, C.L. and Ray, O.S. 2006. *Drugs, Society and Human Behavior*. Columbus, OH: McGraw-Hill.

National Institute on Drug Abuse (NIDA). 2006. *Research Report Series: HIV/AIDS* (NIH Publication Number 06-5760). Washington, D.C.: NIDA.

Rudgley, R. 1993. *Essential Substances*. New York: Kodansha America, Inc.

Search Institute (SEARCH). 2008. *What Are Developmental Assets?* SEARCH Web site. Accessed online November 2008. http://www.search-institute.org/content/what-are-developmental-assets.

Substance Abuse and Mental Health Services Administration (SAMHSA). 2007. *Results from the 2007 National Survey on Drug Use and Health: National Findings*. SAMHSA Web site. Accessed online November 2008. http://www.oas.samhsa.gov/nsduh/2k7nsduh/2k7Results.cfm.

World Health Organization (WHO). 2008a. *Management of Substance Abuse*. WHO Web site. Accessed online November 2008. http://www.who.int/substance_abuse/facts/en/.

_____. 2008b. *Other Psychoactive Substances*. WHO Web site. Accessed online November 2008. http://www.who.int/substance_abuse/facts/psychoactives/en/index.html.

_____. 2008c. *Prevention, Treatment, and Care for Injecting Drug Use (IDU) and Prison*. WHO Web site. Accessed online November 2008. http://www.who.int/hiv/topics/idu/en/index.html.

CHAPTER 16

Prisons and HIV/AIDS

In this chapter, we will examine

- How prisons, simply by their physical structure, give rise to a higher incidence of HIV
- The prevalence of HIV among prison populations
- What is being done to reduce the spread of HIV in prisons

PRISON STRUCTURE

Throughout history people have had to contend with other people behaving in ways deemed detrimental to the health, safety, and survival of the group. Modern societies, of course, send people to prison for various violations of social laws that promote and protect the health, welfare, and safety of the group. If the success of prisons is measured by the number of people housed in penitentiaries at any given time, then prisons have been very successful, especially in the United States, which in 2007 had a national (federal, state, and local jails) prison population of 2,299,116 or roughly 0.7% of the current population (BJS, 2007; CIA, 2008).

The efficacy of prisons as deterrents to further criminal behavior is debatable, because recidivism rates remain high for many crimes (BJS, 1994); what is not debatable, however is the prevalence of HIV/AIDS among prison populations. Indeed, the international data indicate that HIV/AIDS is more of a problem within a prison population than among the general public (WHO, 2008a). Part of the reason for this is the physical structure of prisons. They are buildings with limited space for individuals. This, of course is the intention as prisons were designed as consequences of illegal behavior. In other words, prisons were specifically designed so people would *not* want to commit crimes that would result in them going to prison. Confined in small spaces that are overcrowded, with limited choice of activities, and limited and highly controlled contact with other people are conditions not conducive to high levels of satisfaction and pleasure (Kubzansky, 1961). Indeed, prisons are designed to punish.

The problem with living in close quarters with others is that it increases the likelihood of certain behaviors. Unfortunately, prisons are rife with people who regularly engage in illegal behavior; that's why they are there. The buying, selling, and using of drugs, rape, prostitution, and other forms of sexual assault, and physical violence are some examples of illegal behavior that occur within a prison setting (Beck & Harrison, 2007; WHO, 2005). Considering that HIV is transmitted through contact with bodily fluids, there are many opportunities for persons in prison to come in contact with HIV due to physical space limitations and the increased likelihood of certain risky behaviors.

In sum, prisons have a higher incidence of HIV than the general population due to the persons that are sent there, the kinds of behavior that those people have an increased tendency to engage in, and also due to the physical structure of prisons themselves.

PREVALENCE

As noted, the WHO reports that internationally there are higher rates of HIV infection among prison populations than the general public. This is due in part to a higher number of intravenous drug users (IDUs) that are sent to prison as well as higher rates of infection among the general population in the region of the prison. Their reporting also indicates that while in prison, spread of infection is due to intravenous (IV) drug use, sharing of IV items, sexual activity, tattooing, body piercing, and a high turnover of prisoners (WHO, 2007b; WHO 2008b). As in other locations, women have a lower infection rate than men. Precise measurements of the prevalence of HIV in prison populations are difficult to obtain, but the WHO reports that there have been reports ranging from 0% infection to 50% infection within a prison population (WHO, 2000b). Those that are more likely to become infected use drugs intravenously, abuse alcohol, live in poverty, and come from medically underserved and minority populations (WHO, 2007b).

At the end of 2006 in the United States, there were 21,980 prisoners or 0.46% of the prison population who were HIV-positive or had been diagnosed with AIDS (BJS, 2006). Of these, 19,842 were men and 2,138 were women. There were also 5,674 confirmed AIDS diagnoses and 155 deaths due to AIDS-related causes. At the end of 2006, approximately 1.6% of male and 2.4% of female prisoners nationwide were HIV-positive or diagnosed with AIDS. Texas, New York, and Florida collectively housed 49% of all HIV-positive or AIDS-diagnosed inmates in the country. In addition, these three states also had the highest number of both male and female prisoners that were HIV-positive. National data collected from 2006 support that HIV infection among the U.S. prison population is also higher than among the general public. At the end of 2006, the rate of persons with AIDS was 2.7 times higher among the prison population than among the general public. This was considerably lower than it had been in 1999, when the rate was 4.8 times higher (BJS, 2006).

RESPONSES

Given the above information, the question becomes, how can the spread of HIV be reduced or prevented among prison populations? Not too surprisingly, the answer is through many of the same methods that are used among the general population. We will examine four in particular.

One idea that is somewhat controversial is mandatory testing of prisoners (and in some cases, staff). In some prisons around the world, testing is voluntary, and in others it is mandatory. The WHO recommends against mandatory testing and is in favor of voluntary testing of any prisoners that request testing (WHO, 2007a). Their argument is that mandatory testing is unethical and oftentimes leads to segregating HIV-positive prisoners from the rest of the prison population. Evidence collected by the WHO suggests that both of these measures are counterproductive in reducing the spread of HIV.

The benefit to testing (either voluntary or mandatory) is early identification of HIV infection. This alone could lead to early interventions such as targeted education, personal treatments, and individual prevention efforts. At the end of 2006 in the United States, there were 21 states that tested all prisoners either at admission or while in custody. Forty-seven states offered testing for prisoners that had AIDS symptoms or requested testing. Forty states test if there has been a possibility of exposure, and 16 states test what they define as "high-risk" groups. (See Table 16.1 for a breakdown of all states' requirements by region.)

Another suggestion, far less controversial, is HIV/AIDS education for both prisoners and prison staff. This would include basic information on what HIV is, how it differs from AIDS, how the two are related, how HIV is spread, how it can be prevented. Although data on the overall efficacy of an educational intervention is limited, those data that do exist indicate

Table 16.1 Circumstances under which inmates are tested for the antibody to HIV, 2004

Jurisdiction	All Inmates			High-Risk Groups	Inmate Request	Clinical Indication	Involvement in Incident	Random Sample	Court Order	Other
	Entering	In Custody	Upon Release							
Federal system[1]				X	X	X	X		X	
Northeast										
Connecticut				X	X	X	X		X	
Maine					X	X				
Massachusetts					X					
New Hampshire	X			X	X	X	X			
New Jersey					X	X				
New York				X	X	X	X	X	X	
Pennsylvania				X	X	X	X		X	
Rhode Island	X				X	X	X		X	
Vermont					X	X	X			
Midwest										
Illinois				X	X	X	X		X	
Indiana				X	X	X	X		X	
Iowa	X					X	X			
Kansas				X	X	X	X		X	
Michigan	X				X	X	X		X	
Minnesota				X	X	X	X		X	
Missouri	X		X	X	X	X	X		X	
Nebraska	X				X	X	X		X	
North Dakota	X				X	X			X	
Ohio	X				X	X	X		X	

State	1	2	3	4	5	6	7	8	9	10
South Dakota		×			×	×				
Wisconsin		×		×	×	×				
South										
Alabama		×	×	×	×	×		×		×
Arkansas	×	×		×	×	×	×		×	×
Delaware	×	×		×	×	×				
Florida		×		×	×	×		×		×
Georgia		×		×	×	×	×			
Kentucky		×		×	×					
Louisiana				×	×					
Maryland	×	×		×	×	×				×
Mississippi		×		×	×	×				
North Carolina		×		×	×	×	×			
Oklahoma		×		×	×	×				×
South Carolina	×	×		×	×	×				×
Tennessee		×		×	×	×				
Texas				×	×		×			
Virginia				×	×		×			
West Virginia				×	×					
West										
Arizona		×		×	×	×				
California		×		×	×	×				
Colorado		×		×	×	×				×
Hawaii		×		×	×	×	×			
Idaho		×		×	×	×				×
Montana		×			×	×				

(Continued)

163

Table 16.1 (*Continued*)

Jurisdiction	All Inmates Entering	All Inmates In Custody	Upon Release	High-Risk Groups	Inmate Request	Clinical Indication	Involvement in Incident	Random Sample	Court Order	Other
Nevada		X								
New Mexico					X					X
Oregon				X	X	X	X	X	X	
Utah					X	X	X		X	X
Washington	X			X	X	X	X		X	
Wyoming	X				X	X				X

[1]The Bureau of Prisons tests a random sample of inmates on alternate years. Alaska did not report data on testing.

Bureau of Justice Statistics (BJS). 2008. *HIV in Prisons, 2004.* Accessed online December 2008. http://www.ojp.usdoj.gov/bjs/pub/pdf/hivp04.pdf.

that education does have some positive effect, especially if it is designed and implemented by peers (WHO, 2007a). Education alone is not a necessary and sufficient intervention to stop the spread of HIV within prisons, however. Education can increase the chances of prisoners acting differently due to increased awareness of consequences of their actions, but much more is needed. Unfortunately, one of the fallacies of social intervention work is that education solves everything; it does not. People engage in harmful behavior for many reasons other than lack of knowledge about the consequences of the behavior. It is to other interventions designed to work with people's behavior in mind that we now turn.

As noted, it is well known that sex between prisoners (and some between staff and prisoners) occurs. Sometimes it is coercive, much of it, however, is consensual. In those cases where it is coercive, more work needs to be done by prison staff through differing policies and procedures to reduce the incidence of sexual violence (WHO, 2007c). In the other cases, one recommendation is to provide prisoners with condoms so that when they do engage in sexual intercourse, the potential for exposure to HIV is reduced (WHO, 2007c). It is known that prisoners do use condoms when supplied (although they are generally considered to be contraband) or other barriers that mimic condoms (CDC, 2005b). Although there have been no studies to determine the efficacy of this intervention, there has been information that suggests that when prisons do employ this practice, there has been no increase in violence, no increase in sexual activity, and no increase in drug use; essentially, there have been no reported negative effects of this practice (WHO, 2007a).

Syringe exchange programs (SEP) have been implemented among the general public in countries around the world with varying degrees of success, most of which have been positive. In the United States, the first SEP appeared in 1980; by 2002, there were 184 programs in 36 states that had exchanged over 24 million syringes (CDC, 2005b). Contrary to popular thinking, SEPs have not been found to increase IDUs. These programs remain controversial in the United States, but are more accepted in other countries, notably Europe where the general approach to substance abuse intervention is based on a harm reduction approach. It is no surprise, then, that one approach to reducing HIV/AIDS in prison populations is to implement a SEP within the prison. As noted, this can be seen as a questionable approach, however, as providing persons with clean needles to support their use of illegal drugs is seen by many as enabling the IDU. Similarly, in many jurisdictions in the United States, state and local laws prohibit the distribution and possession of syringes except by prescription (CDC, 2005a).

HARM REDUCTION

The principle of harm reduction does not discount the value of programs that ultimately help drug users defeat their addictions. However, recognizing that becoming drug-free may be a distant goal for many users, harm reduction services are pragmatic measures that seek to minimize certain risks associated with drug use, particularly HIV infection. In other words, if a drug user stops sharing needles with others and uses clean needles provided by a needle exchange program, she or he has reduced the potential harm to self and/or others by not sharing used needles, despite the fact that the intravenous drug use continues. Harm reduction methodologies aim not to endorse or facilitate drug use but to safeguard drug users' human rights and right to dignity.

Harm reduction approaches often involve a dramatic shift in thinking, as for most people, the elimination of drug use from society altogether remains the ultimate, idealistic goal. Some tend to see such harm reduction services as needle exchanges as tacitly encouraging continued drug use and diverting resources away from intervention. However, in actuality, such services help to prevent personal and public health crises, realistically acknowledging that drug use is and will continue to be present in society despite intervention efforts.

Two of the harm reduction services that have proven most effective are needle exchanges and replacement therapy treatment. Other common services include medical referrals, counseling, screening for HIV and other diseases, and health education programs.

Other intervention methods that have been suggested are safer tattooing procedures, narcotic replacement therapies for IDUs injecting heroin or other opiates, drug-free or drug treatment units, and bleach or other sterilization methods to clean syringes between uses. The extent to which each of these approaches are utilized is dependent upon several factors such as funding, public acceptability, ability of prison staff to regulate practices, and other factors.

Managing behavior within a total institution such as a prison is very difficult. Even though it is clear that the prison population has a higher incidence and higher likelihood of becoming HIV infected, solutions are not easily implemented. Change within any organization is difficult. To implement the many ideas on reducing the spread of HIV within prisons would cost money, time, and other resources. Most prisons are under-staffed and underfunded already, so adding additional programming and the staff to accompany that might prove to be a challenge. Similarly, many members of the general public are of the opinion that inmates should not be entitled to additional services. Many see prison as a consequence of bad behavior, a punishment for wrongs committed. As such, it doesn't make sense to provide offenders with more benefits and better services than might be available to the general public. The thinking is that if they become infected with HIV while in prison, it is their own fault and, like imprisonment itself, is just another consequence to bad behavior. As we have seen, however, it is not always as simple as this. Many prisoners are assaulted by others, are victims of rape, are dependent on drugs, and do not always bring bad luck on themselves.

REFERENCES

Beck, A.J., Harrison, P.M. 2007. "Sexual Victimization in State and Federal Prisons Reported by Inmates, 2007." In *Bureau of Justice Statistics Special Report NCJ219414*. Washington, D.C.: BJS.

Bureau of Justice Statistics (BJS). 2006. *HIV in Prisons, 2006*. Washington, D.C.: BJS. BJS Web site. Accessed online November 2008. http://www.ojp.usdoj.gov/bjs/pub/html/hivp/2006/hivp06.htm.

_____. 1994. *Recidivism of Prisoners Released in 1994.*. Washington, D.C.: BJS. BJS Web site. Accessed online November 2008. http://www.ojp.usdoj.gov/bjs/abstract/rpr94.htm.

_____. 2007. *Summary of Findings*. Washington, D.C.: BJS. BJS Web site. Accessed online November 2008. http://www.ojp.usdoj.gov/bjs/prisons.htm.

Centers for Disease Control and Prevention (CDC). 2006. *HIV Transmission Among Male Inmates in a State Prison System—Georgia, 1992–2005*. CDC Web site. Accessed online November 2008. http://www.cdc.gov/mmwr/preview/mmwrhtml/mm5515a1.htm.

_____. 2005a. *State and Local Policies about IDUs' Access to Sterile Syringes*. CDC Web site. Accessed online November 2008. http://www.cdc.gov/idu/facts/AED_IDU_POL.pdf.

_____. 2005b. *Syringe Exchange Programs*. CDC Web site. Accessed online November 2008. http://www.cdc.gov/idu/facts/AED_IDU_SYR.pdf.

Central Intelligence Agency (CIA). 2008. *The World Fact Book*. Washington, D.C.: CIA. CIA Web site. Accessed online November 2008. https://www.cia.gov/library/publications/the-world-factbook/geos/us.html.

Kubzansky, Philip E. 1961. "The Effects of Reduced Environmental Stimulation on Human Behavior: A Review." In *The Manipulation of Human Behavior*. Albert D. Biderman and Herbert Zimmer, eds. New York: John Wiley and Sons, 51–95.

World Health Organization (WHO). 2007a. *Effectiveness of Interventions to Address HIV in Prisons.* Geneva, Switzerland: WHO.

_____. 2007b. *Interventions to Address HIV in Prisons: HIV Care, Treatment, and Support.* Geneva, Switzerland: WHO.

_____. 2007c. *Interventions to Address HIV in Prisons: Prevention of Sexual Transmission.* Geneva, Switzerland: WHO.

_____. 2008a. *Prevention, Treatment and Care for Injecting Drugs Use (IDU) and Prisons.* Geneva, Switzerland: WHO. WHO Web site. Accessed online November 2008. http://www.who.int/hiv/topics/idu/en/index.html.

_____. 2008b. *Prisons.* Geneva, Switzerland: WHO. WHO Web site. Accessed online November 2008. http://www.who.int/hiv/topics/idu/prisons/en/index.html.

_____. 2005. *Status Paper on Prisons, Drugs and Harm Reduction.* Copenhagen, Denmark: WHO.

PART III

Further Information

HIV/AIDS Timeline:
A Chronology
of Significant Events

Date	Medicine & Science	People & Culture	Politics & Activism
1940s	• HIV estimated to have infected humans from primates.		
1950s	• Earliest known cases of AIDS occur; they are not identified as AIDS until decades later.		
1960s–1980	• Early cases of what would come to be known as HIV/AIDS in Central Africa, Canada, Europe, Haiti, and U.S.		
1981	• First report of what would become to be known as AIDS by U.S. Centers for Disease Control on Prevention (CDC) on June 5. This marks the official beginning of the pandemic.	• *New York Times* and National Public Radio run first stories on yet unnamed AIDS.	
1982	• Term "Acquired Immune Deficiency Syndrome" (AIDS) used for the first time. • CDC reports AIDS diagnoses in several infants and young children. • CDC reports first case of possible mother to child transmission. • AIDS reported among hemophiliacs. • First reports of AIDS among Haitians in the U.S. • Ugandan doctors seeing first cases of AIDS.		• Gay Men's Health Crisis founded (NYC). • The Kaposi's Sarcoma Research & Education Foundation (now known as the San Francisco AIDS Foundation) founded. • "San Francisco Model of Care" developed, emphasizing home-based and community services. • The Terry Higgins Trust (later known as the Terrence Higgins Trust), the

1983	• CDC warns about possible problems in the blood supply. • CDC issues recommended precautions for health care workers to avoid AIDS transmission. • First documented U.S. cases of AIDS in heterosexuals; CDC identifies women who have sex with men who have AIDS as a risk group. • Dr. Luc Montagnier and the Institut Pasteur in Paris find virus that will come to be known as HIV. • United Kingdom asks high-risk groups not to donate blood.	• First AIDS candlelight memorial. • Haitian tourism suffers from Haitian association with AIDS.	first AIDS organization in the United Kingdom, formally established. • Congressional hearings on HIV/AIDS. • AIDS Medical Foundation founded (will later become American Foundation for AIDS Research [AmFAR]). • National Association of People with AIDS (NAPWA) formed. • National AIDS Network (NAN) formed. • Federation of AIDS Related Organizations formed. • First U.S. Conference on AIDS, Denver, CO. • U.S. Orphan Drug Act signed. • World Health Organization (WHO) begins global surveillance of AIDS.
1984	• Dr. Robert Gallo at the U.S. National Institutes of Health claims he has identified HIV as cause of AIDS.	• Ryan White, 13-year-old hemophiliac, diagnosed with AIDS. • San Francisco, CA, closes gay bathhouses in the city.	• AIDS Action Council formed. • Zaire's Department of Public Health launches Project SIDA, a national AIDS research program.

Date	Medicine & Science	People & Culture	Politics & Activism
	• CDC identifies reduction in intravenous drug use and needle-sharing as means to prevent HIV transmission. • First needle and syringe exchange program started in Amsterdam, the Netherlands.		
1985	• First HIV antibody test, enzyme linked immunosorbant assay (ELISA), approved by the FDA. • Testing blood products begins (U.S.). • Testing blood products begins (Japan). • Second strain of HIV (HIV-2) discovered in West Africa. • Research confirms condoms prevent spread of HIV. • CDC removes Haitians from list of AIDS high-risk groups. • First reported case of HIV transmission through breast-feeding; recommendations issued for preventing mother-child HIV transmission. • First reported HIV case in China. • WHO definition of AIDS, the Bangui definition, adopted.	• Actor Rock Hudson dies. • Ryan White not allowed to attend school, becomes AIDS advocate. • Larry Kramer's *The Normal Heart* opens in Los Angeles. • First AIDS Walk in U.S. (Los Angeles).	• American Foundation for AIDS Research (AmFAR) founded (previously the AIDS Medical Foundation). • U.S. military begins testing new recruits for HIV. • U.S. President Ronald Reagan uses the word "AIDS" in public for the first time, responding to a reporter's questions. • Project Inform founded. • First International AIDS Conference, Atlanta, GA.

1986

- Lawsuit filed by Pasteur Institute against National Cancer Institute, claiming a share of the royalties from the patented HIV test.
- U.S. Surgeon General Everett Koop publishes a report on AIDS.
- First needle exchange program in U.S. (New Haven, CT).
- AZT clinical trials begin.
- First UK needle exchange program, Dundee.
- First HIV cases reported in India.
- Cuba begins to screen blood donors for HIV.

- U.S. hospital accused of illegal civil rights violation in case of fired nurse with AIDS.

- Congress established funding ($47 million) to establish the AIDS Clinical Trials Group (ACTG).
- World Health Organization founds Global Programme on AIDS.
- Second International AIDS Conference, Paris, France.

1987

- First anti-HIV drug, AZT, approved by the FDA; the cost is $12,000 annually.
- First Western Blot blood test kit approved by the FDA; screens for HIV antibodies.
- First human testing of HIV vaccine sanctioned by the FDA.
- FDA publishes regulations requiring HIV antibodies screening of all blood and plasma collected in the U.S.

- Michael Bennett, Broadway director, dies.
- Liberace, entertainer, dies.
- Ray family home burned by arsonist, Florida (family with 3 HIV+ hemophiliac siblings).
- Randy Shilts publishes *And the Band Played On.*
- First AIDS-related public service announcements from the CDC, "America Responds to AIDS."
- AIDS Memorial Quilt displayed on the National Mall in Washington, D.C.

- AIDS Coalition to Unleash Power (ACT-UP) founded in NYC.
- President Ronald Reagan delivers his only "major speech" on AIDS.
- Association of Nurses in AIDS Care founded.
- U.S. policy bans entry of HIV+ immigrants and travelers.
- First National Conference on AIDS and communities of color held by CDC.
- National Black Leadership Commission on AIDS formed.

Date	Medicine & Science	People & Culture	Politics & Activism
	• First infection with HIV-2 reported in the U.S. • CDC publishes precautions that became Universal Precautions (UP), more issued in 1991. • Treatment Investigational New Drug (INDs) category established by FDA to accelerate drug approval process. • Researcher Dr. Peter Duesberg publishes article challenging HIV/AIDS link. • First case of HIV recorded in Russia. • WHO confirms HIV can be passed from mother-to-child through breastfeeding. • Agreement reached that Pasteur Institute and U.S. DHHS would share profits from HIV antibody test patent.	• U.S. Central Intelligence Agency (CIA) predicts devastating impact of AIDS in Africa. • Princess Diana visits AIDS ward and touches patients. • Australian "Grim Reaper" education campaign launched.	• National Minority AIDS Council formed. • National Task Force on AIDS Prevention formed. • Helms Amendment passed by U.S. Congress that prohibits AIDS education funding encouraging or promoting homosexuality. • World Health Organization launches Global Program on AIDS. • UN General Assembly debates AIDS—first disease ever debated on that floor. • Third International AIDS Conference, Washington, D.C.
1988	• Importation of unapproved HIV/AIDS treatments for personal use approved by the FDA. • FDA implemented regulations designed to expedite approval of new therapies.	• "Understanding AIDS," booklet by Surgeon General C. Everett Koop mailed to 110 million U.S. households.	• Discrimination against federal workers with HIV banned in U.S. • ACT-UP demonstrates at FDA headquarters for faster HIV drug approval process; new regulations announced days later.

	• Office of AIDS Research (OAR) established by the National Institutes of Health. • AIDS Clinical Trials group (ACTG) established by the National Institutes of Health. • Needle exchange programs (NEPs) established, Tacoma, WA, New York, NY, and San Francisco, CA.			• Pediatric AIDS Foundation founded. • International AIDS Society formed. • First World AIDS Day, World Health Organization, (December 1). • Fourth International AIDS Conference, Stockholm, Sweden.
1989	• First HIV-1 antigen diagnostic kit approved by FDA.	• Alvin Ailey, choreographer, dies. • Amanda Blake, actress, dies. • Esteban Dejesus, World Boxing Championship lightweight champion, dies. • Robert Mapplethorpe, photographer, dies. • Tim Richmond, NASCAR driver, dies; his HIV+ status not confirmed until 1996. • National Endowment for the Arts withdraws grant from a NYC gallery exhibit on AIDS. • AIDS Memorial Quilt nominated for Nobel Peace Prize.	• National Commission on AIDS issues first report. • Fifth International AIDS Conference, Montreal, Canada.	
1990	• CDC reports possible case of transmission of HIV from dentist David Acer to patient Kimberly Bergalis.	• Halston, American fashion designer, dies. • Keith Haring, artist, dies.		• U.S. Congress enacts Ryan White Care Act, funded at $220 million. • Americans With Disabilities Act (ADA) enacted by Congress.

Date	Medicine & Science	People & Culture	Politics & Activism
	• Needle exchange in NYC shut down. • Millions in compensation announced for HIV-infected hemophiliacs and survivors in the United Kingdom.	• Ryan White, hemophiliac, teen AIDS activist, dies.	• AEGIS founded. • First National Conference on Women and AIDS, Boston, MA. • Sixth International AIDS Conference, San Francisco, CA.
1991	• Kimberly Bergalis testifies before Congress, asking health care workers to be forced to submit to HIV tests. • Videx (didanosine, ddI) approved for treatment of AIDS by FDA. • First combination HIV-1 and HIV-2 antibody test licensed. • HIV+ hemophiliacs in France sue medical and government officials accusing blood transfusion centers use of infected blood.	• 10th anniversary of first published report of what would come to be known as AIDS. • Earvin "Magic" Johnson reveals he is HIV+. • Kimberly Bergalis dies. • Freddy Mercury, lead singer in rock band "Queen," dies. • Red Ribbon becomes symbol for HIV/AIDS.	• Housing Opportunities for Persons with AIDS (HOPWA) program authorized by the National Affordable Housing Act of 1990 (revised in 1992). • International Council of AIDS Service Organizations (ICASO) forms. • Seventh International AIDS Conference, Florence, Italy.
1992	• First rapid HIV test (SUDS HIV-1) approved by FDA. • FDA approves zalcitabine (ddC) for use in combination with AZT resulting in first successful combination therapy.	• Ricky Ray, teenage hemophiliac, dies. • Robert Reed, actor, dies. • Arthur Ashe, tennis star, announces he has AIDS. • First drive-up "Condom Hut" opens (Cranston, Rhode Island). • Four French health care officials tried on tainted blood charges; 3 convicted, 2 imprisoned.	• Indian government allocates $100 million to fight growing rates of HIV. • Eighth International AIDS Conference, Amsterdam (moved from Boston due to immigration ban).

1993

- Reality Female Condom approved for use by FDA.
- CDC revises definition of AIDS.
- Drug-resistant strains of HIV reported.
- Arthur Ashe dies.
- Katrina Haslip, advocate for imprisoned women with AIDS, dies.
- Rudolf Nureyev, ballet dancer, dies.
- Tony Kushner's *Angels in America* wins Pulitzer and Tony Award.
- *Philadelphia* released.
- HIV+ foreigners banned from obtaining U.S. citizenship or visas.
- White House Office of National AIDS Policy (ONAP) established.
- First annual AIDSWatch lobbies Congress for AIDS funding.
- Ninth International AIDS Conference, Berlin, Germany.

1994

- First oral HIV test, Orasure, (first nonblood-based collection kit) approved by the FDA.
- AZT recommended to reduce mother-to-infant HIV transmission.
- FDA approves polyurethane condom for use by individuals who are allergic to latex.
- John Curry, Olympic figure skater, dies.
- Elizabeth Glaser, Pediatric AIDS advocate, dies.
- Dack Rambo, actor, dies.
- Randy Shilts, author of *And the Band Played On*, dies.
- Pedro Zamora, activist/educator, appears on MTV's *The Real World*; dies.
- Tom Hanks wins Oscar for *Philadelphia*.
- CDC launches series of AIDS ads focusing on condom use.
- President Clinton asks U.S. Surgeon General Jocelyn Elders to resign after controversial remarks about content of sex education at a World AIDS Day conference.
- 18 members of the National Task Force on AIDS Drug Development announced.
- Tenth International AIDS Conference, Yokohama, Japan.

Date	Medicine & Science	People & Culture	Politics & Activism
1995	• First protease inhibitor class anti-HIV drug, Saquinavir, approved for U.S. use. • CDC issues first guidelines for prevention of AIDS-related opportunistic infections. • CDC announces AIDS has become leading cause of death among adults age 25–44. • Blood donor criteria revised by FDA excluding prisoners from donating blood, blood components, and plasma for 12 months from last date of incarceration. • U.S. admits Montagnier at Institut Pasteur, not Robert Gallo at NIH, who discovered HIV.	• Glenn Burke, professional baseball player, dies. • Eric "Eazy-E" Wright, rapper, dies. • Greg Louganis, Olympic gold medal diver, reveals that he has AIDS.	• Presidential Advisory Council on HIV/AIDS established by President Clinton. • First White House Summit on AIDS held. • First U.S. National HIV Testing Day. • WHO Global Programme on AIDS discontinued, replaced by the Joint United Nations Program on HIV/AIDS (UNAIDS).
1996	• First nonnucleoside reverse transcriptase inhibitor (NNRTI), Viramune (nevirapine), approved. • First viral load test approved to measure level of HIV in the body and gauge treatment effects. • FDA approves first home HIV test kit (Confide HIV Testing System); it becomes available and can be purchased over-the-counter (OTC).	• Peter Adair, filmmaker, dies. • Tommy Morrison, heavyweight boxer, announces he is HIV+. • Musical *Rent* moves to Broadway and wins major awards. • National AIDS Memorial Grove Act approved by Congress, President. • Complete AIDS Memorial Quilt displayed in Washington DC for the final time (October 11–13).	• Ryan White Care Act reauthorized by Congress. • Congress passes, then later repeals, a measure to honorably discharge all HIV+ military personnel. • President Clinton announces first White House AIDS strategy. • Joint United Nations Program on HIV/AIDS (UNAIDS) begins operation.

1997

- First HIV-1 antigen test kit, Coulter HIV-1 p24 Antigen Assay, approved by FDA.
- First urine HIV test approved by FDA.
- AIDS researcher Dr. David Ho named *TIME* magazine's Man of the Year.
- International AIDS Vaccine Initiative (IAVI) formed.
- Brazil begins distribution nationwide of free HIV combination drugs.
- Eleventh International AIDS Conference, Vancouver, Canada.
- CDC reports a case of probable transmission of HIV through deep kissing.
- FDA requires labeling of latex condoms with an expiration date.
- Number of newly diagnosed AIDS cases in U.S. drops for the first time since epidemic began, credited to advances in medication.
- U.S. President Clinton calls for an HIV vaccine in 10 years.
- FDA Modernization Act enacted by Congress.

1998

- Donna Shalala, Secretary of the Department of Health and Human Services (DHHS), announces that needle exchange programs lessen spread of HIV without increasing drug use.
- South African AIDS activist Gugu Dlamini beaten to death by neighbors after revealing on television she was HIV+.
- U.S. Supreme Court rules that HIV+ individuals, not only those with AIDS, are covered under the Americans with Disabilities Act.
- Minority AIDS Initiative formed, $150 million in funding by Congress.

Date	Medicine & Science	People & Culture	Politics & Activism
	• Drug-resistant HIV strains reported. • First Phase III (large scale) clinical vaccine trial begins by company AIDSvax. • FDA approved Glyde Dam Lollyes dental dams for use during oral sex. • First national guidelines on use of ARVs issued by DHHS.		• Ricky Ray Hemophilia Relief Fund Act of 1998 enacted by Congress. • Twelfth International AIDS Conference, Geneva, Switzerland.
1999	• Human vaccine trial begins in Thailand. • Uganda begins door-to-door rapid HIV testing.	• Reggie Williams, founder of the National AIDS Task Force on AIDS Prevention, dies. • American Medical Association advocates handing out condoms in schools. • Dr. Richard Schmidt sentenced to 50 years in prison on conviction of injecting his former lover with HIV infected blood. • China broadcasts first televised condom ad; the ad was subsequently banned.	• Congressional hearing on HIV/AIDS in Hispanic communities. • Amsterdam Statement by international health organizations calls for affordable drugs. • Kenyan President Daniel arap Moi orders establishment of a National AIDS Control Council
2000	• Durban Declaration released to press (July 1) signed by scientists/physicians from around the world who affirm HIV is cause of AIDS.	• Reverend Jesse Jackson publicly takes oral HIV test to focus on increasing number of infected African Americans. • United Nations Security Council and U.S. both identify AIDS as threat to global security.	• Ryan White Comprehensive AIDS Resources Emergency (CARE) Act reauthorized by Congress. • Global AIDS Program (GAP) formed by CDC.

2001	• CDC reports new HIV infections growing twice as fast in 50+ age group than among younger age groups.
	• DHHS review panel confirms latex condoms effective against HIV transmission.
	• FDA licenses first Nucleic Acid Test (NAT) system to screen plasma HIV and Hepatitis C.
	• 20th anniversary of first published report of what would come to be known as AIDS.
	• FDA issues warning letter to pharmaceutical companies that optimistic tone of HIV drug ads is misleading.
	• China acknowledges growing AIDS problem.
	• Colin Powell calls HIV/AIDS a threat to national security.
	• Former Japanese health minister found guilty for not stopping sale of untreated blood products.
	• Global AIDS and Tuberculosis Relief Act of 2000, up to $600 million authorized.
	• Accelerating Access Initiative formed to provide drugs to poor nations.
	• Millennium Vaccine Initiative created.
	• Thirteenth International AIDS Conference, Durban, South Africa.
	• First Annual National Black HIV/AIDS Awareness Day in U.S.
	• United Nations General Assembly Special Session (UNGASS) held on AIDS.
	• United Nations Declaration of Commitment on HIV/AIDS signed at UNGASS by 189 countries.
	• World Trade Organization ministers agree on Doha (Qatar) Declaration aimed at making generic drugs more available to poor nations.
2002	• First rapid finger prick test approved by FDA.
	• Botswana government institutes free ARV drug distribution.
	• First Brazilian HIV prevention campaign targeting gay men.
	• India posts world's largest number of AIDS orphans.
	• Abstinence-only education programs begin to be promoted by the Bush administration.

Date	Medicine & Science	People & Culture	Politics & Activism
		• Portugal posts highest rate of HIV infection among European Union nations. • Kami, HIV+ character, joins cast of South African version of *Sesame Street*. • Ukraine becomes first European nation with 1% of adult population HIV+. • WHO funds first HIV/AIDS survey in Afghanistan.	• USAID announces ABC approach to prevention (**A**bstinence, **B**eing faithful, and **C**ondom use). • Global Fund to Fight AIDS, Tuberculosis, and Malaria begins operation. • Fourteenth International AIDS Conference, Barcelona, Spain.
2003	• First federal clinical guide released by the U.S. DHHS. • Advancing HIV Prevention (AHP) announced by CDC, refocusing prevention efforts on those already infected. • VAXgen confirms AIDSvax clinical trials have not produced a viable vaccine. • Fuzeon, the first fusion inhibitor class HIV drug, approved by the FDA for those who have developed resistance to other ARVs.	• *Angels in America* airs on HBO. • Swaziland has highest rate of HIV infection in the world. • Manslaughter charges filed by Treatment Action Campaign (TAC) against several South African government ministers for not providing access to ARV drugs. • Wen Jiabao, Chinese premier, handshake with AIDS patient is broadcast.	• First Annual National Latino AIDS Awareness Day in U.S. • President's Emergency Plan for AIDS Relief (PEPFAR) announced by U.S. President George Bush—5 year, $15 billion effort. • HIV drug makers lower price of ARVs in poor countries. • UN World Food Programme shifts southern Africa humanitarian aid programs toward HIV/AIDS. • World Health Organization announces "3 × 5 Initiative" (to treat 3 million people by 2005). • Chinese government announces "Four Frees and One Care" series of HIV initiatives.

2004

- FDA approves first generic HIV drug.
- FDA approves Multispot HIV-1/HIV-2 Rapid Test.
- FDA approves, OraQuick Rapid HIV-1 Antibody Test, first rapid test to use oral fluid.

- HIV in adult film industry impacts production and gains government attention.
- Malawi President Bakili Muluzi announces his brother died from AIDS.
- United Nations report addresses growing problem of AIDS in Eastern Europe and the former Soviet Union.
- South African Treatment Action Campaign and leader, Zackie Achmat, jointly nominated for Nobel Peace Prize.

- The Bill and Melinda Gates Foundation awards $60 million for research and development of microbicides.
- First funding begins for PEPFAR.
- Call by leaders of powerful Group of Eight (G8) nations for "Global HIV Vaccine Enterprise".
- South Africa begins new ARV treatment program.
- Fifteenth International AIDS Conference, Bangkok, Thailand.

2005

- FDA changes allow non-U.S. manufacturers to produce generic HIV drugs for PEPFAR.
- Four generic forms of AZT go on sale in the U.S. when the patent expires.
- Patient infected with HIV by her HIV+ obstetrician during a cesarean section (Spain).

- Video version of *Rent* released.
- Nelson Mandela announces his eldest son Makgatho died of AIDS.

- First U.S. National Asian and Pacific Islander HIV/AIDS Awareness Day.
- Russian President Vladimir Putin acknowledges Russian AIDS problem and pledges financial resources.
- World Health Organization, UNAIDS, the United States Government, and the Global Fund to

Date	Medicine & Science	People & Culture	Politics & Activism
			Fight AIDS, Tuberculosis and Malaria hold press conference on efforts to increase access to antiretroviral treatment.
			• G8 Summit and World Economic Forum both include focus on HIV/AIDS in Africa.
2006	• FDA requires warnings on all latex condoms ("Condoms greatly reduce, but do not eliminate the risk of pregnancy and HIV infection when used correctly during sexual intercourse.").	• U2 rock star Bono announces "Product RED" commercial brand to support Global Fund.	• First U.S. Nation Women and Girls HIV/AIDS Awareness Day.
		• The Lancet and The Independent, a British medical journal and newspaper, publish special Product RED editions.	• Ryan White Care Act reauthorized by U.S. Congress for third time; renamed Ryan White AIDS Treatment Modernization Act of 2006.
	• FDA approves first one-a-day HIV treatment, Altripa.		• First Global AIDS Week (February 27–March 3).
	• CDC recommends routine HIV screening for all people ages 13–64, yearly screening for those in high-risk categories.		• World Health Organization (WHO) and the Joint United Nations Programme on HIV/AIDS shows "3 x 5 Initiative" fell short.
	• WHO warns about an extremely drug-resistant strain of tuberculosis.		• UNAIDS comprehensive report on global epidemic.
			• Moscow hosts Far Eastern European and Central Asian AIDS Conference.
			• Sixteenth International AIDS Conference, Toronto Canada.

| 2007 | • Updated antiretroviral treatment guidelines issued by U.S. DHHS.
• FDA approves maraviroc (Selzentry) and raltegravir (Isentress) for those with drug resistant viral strain.
• WHO and UNAIDS recommend consideration of male circumcision as part of HIV prevention efforts.
• Large microbicide study halted after poor results.
• Large vaccine trial halted after poor results.
• Counterfeit ARVs flood Zimbabwe. | • Official New York City and Washington DC condoms unveiled as public health measure.
• President Jammeh of The Gambia announces falsely he has found AIDS cure. | • First annual Native American HIV/AIDS Awareness Day.
• Institute of Medicine (IOM) report praises, but urges changes in, PEPFAR.
• International HIV/AIDS Implementers Meeting, Kigali, Rwanda. |
| 2008 | • CDC issues increased estimates (from 40,000 to 56,300) of annual new HIV infections in the United States.
• FC2, a lower-cost, second-generation female condom approved for use by FDA. | • Luc Montaginer and Francoise Barre-Sinoussi win Nobel Prize in Physiology and Medicine for discovery of HIV. | • Global Leadership Against HIV/AIDS, Tuberculosis, and Malaria Reauthorization Act of 2008 signed by President Bush; this PEPFAR reauthorization repeals 1993 law preventing HIV+ immigrants and visitors to U.S.
• International HIV/AIDS Implementers Meeting, Kampala, Uganda.
• WHO, UNAIDS, and UNICEF report significant increase over past 4 years of ART treatment in low/middle income countries. |

187

Date	Medicine & Science	People & Culture	Politics & Activism
2009	• Washington, D.C., Health Department report revels higher rate of HIV than West Africa. • German physicians report that after a bone marrow transplant in an HIV+ leukemia patient, the patient no longer shows signs of HIV infection. • World Health Organization reports that a quarter of tuberculosis deaths are HIV-related.	• Obama Administration, through CDC, launches "Act Against AIDS" national public health campaign. • Pope Benedict XVI visits Africa, emphasizes abstinence and says that condoms can "increase the problem" of HIV/AIDS.	• Seventeenth International AIDS Conference, Mexico City, Mexico. • United Nations marks International Women's Day, highlighting link between violence against women and girls, and HIV.

REFERENCES

AEGIS, AIDS Education Global Information System. No date. "So Little Time. . .
    An AIDS History." AEGIS Web site. Accessed online August 2008. http://
    www.aegis.com/topics/timeline/default.asp.
AIDS Action. "Keeping Time: Social and Governmental Developments in HIV."
    AIDS Action Web site. Accessed online November 2008. http://www.
    aidsaction.org/timeline/index.htm.
AVERTing HIV and AIDS (Avert). "'The History of AIDS' timelines. " AVERT
    Web site. Accessed online November 2008. http://www.avert.org/his81_
    86.htm.
Frontline. "Timeline: 25 Years of AIDS." The Age of AIDS PBS Web site.
    Accessed online August 2008. http://www.pbs.org/wgbh/pages/frontline/
    aids/cron/.
The Kaiser Family Foundation (KFF). "The Global HIV/AIDS Timeline." KFF
    Web site. Accessed online November 2008. http://www.kff.org/hivaids/
    timeline/hivtimeline.cfm.
San Francisco AIDS Foundation. "HIV/AIDS Timeline. Milestones in the Battle
    Against AIDS." SFAF Web site. Accessed online November 2008. http://
    www.sfaf.org/custom/timeline.aspx?l=en&y=0000&t=all.
Stine, Gerald J. 2009. *AIDS Update 2008*. Boston: McGraw-Hill.
U.S. Food and Drug Administration (FDA). "FDA HIV/AIDS Time Line—A
    Chronology of Significant Events." FDA Web site. Accessed online 2008.
    http://www.fda.gov/oashi/aids/miles81.html.
Wessner, David. No date. "HIV/AIDS in Popular Culture" Timeline. Davidson
    College, David Wenner Web site. Accessed online October 2008.
    http://www.bio.davidson.edu/projects/aidspopculture/.

APPENDIX B

Primary Documents

PNEUMOCYSTIS PNEUMONIA— LOS ANGELES

The CDC's first published report on what would come to be known as AIDS.

In the period October 1980–May 1981, 5 young men, all active homosexuals, were treated for biopsy-confirmed *Pneumocystis carinii* pneumonia at 3 different hospitals in Los Angeles, California. Two of the patients died. All 5 patients had laboratory-confirmed previous or current cytomegalovirus (CMV) infection and candidal mucosal infection. Case reports of these patients follow.

Patient 1: A previously healthy 33-year-old man developed *P. carinii* pneumonia and oral mucosal candidiasis in March 1981 after a 2-month history of fever associated with elevated liver enzymes, leukopenia, and CMV viruria. The serum complement-fixation CMV titer in October 1980 was 256; in May 1981 it was 32. The patient's condition deteriorated despite courses of treatment with trimethoprim-sulfamethoxazole (TMP/SMX), pentamidine, and acyclovir. He died May 3, and postmortem examination showed residual *P. carinii* and CMV pneumonia, but no evidence of neoplasia.

Patient 2: A previously healthy 30-year-old man developed *p. carinii* pneumonia in April 1981 after a 5-month history of fever each day and of elevated liver-function tests, CMV viruria, and documented seroconversion to CMV, i.e., an acute-phase titer of 16 and a convalescent-phase titer of 28 in anticomplement immunofluorescence tests. Other features of his illness included leukopenia and mucosal candidiasis. His pneumonia responded to a course of intravenous TMP/SMX, but, as of the latest reports, he continues to have a fever each day.

Patient 3: A 30-year-old man was well until January 1981 when he developed esophageal and oral candidiasis that responded to Amphotericin B treatment. He was hospitalized in February 1981 for *P. carinii* pneumonia that responded to TMP/SMX. His esophageal candidiasis recurred after the pneumonia was diagnosed, and he was again given Amphotericin B. The CMV complement-fixation titer in March 1981 was 8. Material from an esophageal biopsy was positive for CMV.

Patient 4: A 29-year-old man developed *P. carinii* pneumonia in February 1981. He had had Hodgkin's disease 3 years earlier, but had been successfully treated with radiation therapy alone. He did not improve after being given intravenous TMP/SMX and corticosteroids and died in March. Postmortem examination showed no evidence of Hodgkin's disease, but *P. carinii* and CMV were found in lung tissue.

Patient 5: A previously healthy 36-year-old man with clinically diagnosed CMV infection in September 1980 was seen in April 1981 because of a 4-month history of fever, dyspnea, and cough. On admission he was found to have *P. carinii* pneumonia, oral candidiasis, and CMV retinitis. A complement-fixation CMV titer in April 1981 was 128. The patient has been treated with 2 short courses of TMP/SMX that have been limited because of a sulfa-induced neutropenia. He is being treated for candidiasis with topical nystatin.

The diagnosis of *Pneumocystis* pneumonia was confirmed for all 5 patients antemortem by closed or open lung biopsy. The patients did not know each other and had no known common contacts or knowledge of sexual partners who had had similar illnesses. Two of the 5 reported having frequent homosexual contacts with various partners. All 5 reported using inhalant drugs, and 1 reported parenteral drug abuse. Three patients had profoundly depressed *in vitro* proliferative responses to mitogens and antigens. Lymphocyte studies were not performed on the other 2 patients.

Reported by M.S. Gottlieb, MD, H.M. Schanker, MD, P.T. Fan, MD, A. Saxon, MD, J.D. Weisman, DO, Div of Clinical Immunology-Allergy; Dept of Medicine, UCLA School of Medicine; I. Pozalski, MD, Cedars-Mt. Sinai Hospital, Los Angeles; Field Services Div., Epidemiology Program Office, CDC.

Editorial Note

Pneumocystis pneumonia in the United States is almost exclusively limited to severely immunosuppressed patients (1). The occurrence of pneumocystosis in these 5 previously healthy individuals without a clinically apparent underlying immunodeficiency is unusual. The fact that these patients were all homosexuals suggests an association between some aspect of a homosexual lifestyle or disease acquired through sexual contact and *Pneumocystis* pneumonia in this population. All 5 patients described in this report had laboratory-confirmed CMV disease or virus shedding within 5 months of the diagnosis of *Pneumocystis* pneumonia. CMV infection has been shown to induce transient abnormalities of *in vitro* cellular-immune function in otherwise healthy human hosts (2, 3). Although all 3 patients tested had abnormal cellular-immune function, no definitive conclusion regarding the role of CMV infection in these 5 cases can be reached because of the lack of published data on cellular-immune function in healthy homosexual males with and without CMV antibody. In 1 report, 7 (3.6%) of 194 patients with pneumocystosis also had CMV infection: 40 (21%) of the same group had at least

1 other major concurrent infection (1). A high prevalence of CMV infections among homosexual males was recently reported: 179 (94%) had CMV viruria; rates for 101 controls of similar age who were reported to be exclusively hetero-sexual were 54% for seropositivity and zero fro viruria (4). In another study of 64 males, 4 (6.3%) had positive tests for CMV in semen, but none had CMV recovered from urine. Two of the 4 reported recent homosexual contacts. These findings suggest not only that virus shedding may be more readily detected in seminal fluid than urine, but also that seminal fluid may be an important vehicle of CMV transmission (5).

All the above observations suggest the possibility of a cellular-immune dys-function related to a common exposure that predisposes individuals to oppor-tunistic infections such as pneumocystosis and candidiasis. Although the role of CMV infection in the pathogenesis of pneumocystosis remains unknown, the possibility of *P. carinii* infection must be carefully considered in a differential diagnosis for previously healthy homosexual males with dyspnea and pneumonia.

REFERENCES

1. Walzer PD, Perl DP, Krogstad DJ, Rawson G, Schultz MG. *Pneumocystis carinii* Pneumonia in the United States. Epidemiologic, Diagnostic, and Clinical Features. Ann Intern Med 1974; 80: 83–93.
2. Rinaldo CR, Jr, Black PH, Hirsh MS. Interaction of cytomegalovirus with leukocytes from patients with mononucleosis due to cytomegalovirus. J Infect Dis 1977; 136: 667–78.
3. Rinaldo CR, Jr, Carney WP, Richter BS, Black PH, Hirsh MS. Mechanisms of Immunosuppression in Cytomegaloviral Mononucleosis. J Infect Dis 1980; 141: 488–95.
4. Drew WL, Mintz L, Miner RC, Sands M, Ketterer B. Prevalence of Cytomegalovirus Infection in Homosexual Men. J Infect Dis 1981; 143: 188–92.
5. Lang DJ, Kummer JF. Cytomegalovirus in Semen: Observations in Selected Populations. J Infect Dis 1975; 132: 472–73.

Source

Morbidity and Mortality Weekly Report (MMWR). June 5, 1981: 30(21); 1–3. Accessed online September 2008. http://www.cdc.gov/mmwr/Preview/mmwrhtml/june_5.htm.

TWENTY-FIVE YEARS OF HIV/AIDS— UNITED STATES, 1981-2006

The CDC reports on the first quarter century of the HIV/AIDS pandemic.

On June 5, 1981, *MMWR* published a report of *Pneumocystis carinii* pneumonia in five previously healthy young men in Los Angeles, California (*1*). These cases were later recognized as the first reported cases of acquired immunodeficiency syndrome (AIDS) in the United States. Since that time, this disease has become one of the greatest public health challenges both nationally and globally. Human immunodeficiency virus (HIV) and AIDS have claimed the lives of more than 22 million persons worldwide, including more than 500,000 persons in the United States.

In 2006, more than 1 million persons are living with HIV/AIDS in the United States, and an estimated 40,000 new HIV infections are expected to occur this year (*2*). Since the beginning of the epidemic, countless persons and organizations, inside and outside of government, have mobilized to prevent and treat this disease. These efforts have been enhanced by the commitment and involvement of those living with HIV/AIDS. At this milestone marking the 25th year of AIDS, one way to recognize those persons who have died and those who have been affected by this epidemic is to accelerate the development of measures for preventing HIV transmission.

Successes in HIV Prevention

CDC's overarching HIV-prevention goal is to reduce the number of new HIV infections and to eliminate racial and ethnic disparities by the promotion of HIV counseling, testing, and referral and by encouraging HIV prevention among both persons living with HIV and those at high risk for contracting the virus (*3*).

The decrease in mother-to-child (perinatal) HIV transmission is a public health achievement in HIV prevention in the United States. The number of infants infected with HIV through perinatal transmission has decreased from 1,650 during the early- to mid-1990s to 144–236 in 2002 (*4*). This decline is attributed to multiple interventions, including routine voluntary HIV testing of pregnant women, the use of rapid HIV tests at delivery for women of unknown HIV status, and the use of antiretroviral therapy by HIV-infected women during pregnancy and by infants after birth.

Widespread availability and use of diagnostic and screening tests for HIV infection to promote individual knowledge of HIV serostatus and to ensure the safety of the nation's blood supply has been another success. Since the mid-1980s, blood donor screening methods and testing technology have steadily improved; today, with nucleic acid testing, the risk for HIV transmission is estimated at as low as one per 2 million blood donations (*5*). Widespread HIV testing promotion and uptake have resulted in approximately 50% of persons aged 15–44 years in the United States reporting that they have had an HIV test (*6*), with a high proportion of those at increased risk (e.g., men who have sex with men [MSM] and injection-drug users) reporting having an HIV test during the preceding year (6, 7).

National HIV-prevention initiatives have been supported by HIV-prevention programs of state and local health departments, community-based organizations, and other partners (8). Prevention interventions, including drug treatment programs, peer outreach, and risk reduction, have contributed to a steady decline in new HIV/AIDS diagnoses among injection-drug users in 35 areas with HIV reporting, from an estimated 8,048 in 2001 to 5,962 in 2004 (9). Another prevention success has been the diffusion of evidence-based effective behavioral interventions (DEBIs) for primary and secondary HIV prevention among persons, small groups, and communities (3). These interventions help to ensure that those persons at greatest risk for HIV transmission or acquisition are able to obtain intensive support to reduce risk behaviors and adopt protective strategies for their health and the health of their partners.

Remaining Challenges

Despite these successes, several challenges remain. HIV/AIDS continues to be a leading cause of illness and death in the United States. An estimated 252,000–312,000 HIV-infected persons in the United States are unaware of their HIV infection (2). Not only are they at high risk for transmitting HIV to others, but they are much less likely to take advantage of effective medical treatments.

Certain subpopulations remain at increased risk. MSM account for approximately 45% of newly reported HIV/AIDS diagnoses and nearly 54% of cumulative AIDS diagnoses (10, 11). A recent survey indicated that in several large U.S. cities, approximately one in four MSM surveyed in social venues is infected with HIV, and nearly 50% of MSM are unaware of their HIV infections (12). Moreover, young MSM were least likely to know they were infected, and MSM from racial/ethnic minority populations consistently demonstrated higher prevalence than white MSM. Annual HIV incidence among MSM is high, ranging from 1.2% to 8.0% (12). Racial and ethnic minority communities also are disproportionately affected by HIV/AIDS (13). During 2001–2004, in 35 areas with HIV reporting, 51% of all new HIV/AIDS diagnoses were among blacks, who account for approximately 13% of the U.S. population (14). Of these, 11% (12,650) of HIV/AIDS diagnoses in men were in black men who were infected through heterosexual contact, and 54% (23,820) of HIV/AIDS diagnoses in women were in black women infected through heterosexual contact. Today, women account for approximately one quarter of all new HIV/AIDS diagnoses and, in 2002, HIV infection was the leading cause of death for black women aged 25–34 years.

A scaling up of the diffusion of effective behavioral interventions (e.g., DEBIs) is required; however, limitations exist in CDC's ability to meet current training and technical assistance needs, as well as states' abilities to implement them widely. Other gaps include the lack of data regarding the effectiveness of adapting DEBIs to all at-risk populations (15). In many locales, the community-level workforce might be weakened by attrition, fatigue, and inadequate program skills (*15,16*). Changing public perceptions of HIV/AIDS in the United States, coupled with the widespread availability of highly active antiretroviral treatment, has led to the widespread belief that AIDS is no longer a problem or a severe disease in the United States (*17*). Although 26% of persons in the United States consider AIDS as a top health concern for the nation (second only to cancer [35%]), the proportion who see it as the number one health problem has declined during the past few years (*18*). Complacency, stigma, and discrimination persist and all decrease motivation among persons and communities to adopt risk-reduction behaviors, get tested for HIV, and access prevention and treatment services (*19*).

New Strategies

Despite these challenges, substantial opportunities remain to enhance and demonstrate the effectiveness of HIV-prevention measures. New strategies will need to be combined with a scaling up of traditionally effective interventions that are tailored for local epidemiology and context to maximize public health impact despite resource constraints.

Partnerships

Eliminating HIV/AIDS in the United States cannot be achieved by any single agency or group, but will require public health partnerships comprising persons, communities, agencies, and the private sector. Strong partnerships are especially important to address stigma and discrimination and to promote greater acceptance of those living with HIV/AIDS. Religious and business communities and correctional and mental health services all need to be part of a national mobilization in the prevention of HIV transmission (*20*). Improved collaboration across government agencies is also required to provide a unified public health infrastructure dedicated to research, prevention, treatment, care, and rehabilitative services for persons affected by HIV/AIDS.

Increased Access to Voluntary HIV Testing

For the estimated quarter of a million persons living with HIV who are unaware of their HIV infection, testing is the gateway to lifesaving treatment. Persons who know they are infected with HIV are more likely to take steps to prevent themselves from transmitting the virus to others (*21*). To reduce the number of persons with undiagnosed HIV infections, a sustained expansion of access to and uptake of HIV testing will be required. This reduction can be achieved by making voluntary HIV testing a routine part of medical care, reducing the barriers to HIV testing, and ensuring easy access to new rapid HIV tests that, in many jurisdictions, can be performed by trained persons who are not clinicians (*22–24*).

Prevention Messages Focused on Both HIV-Positive and HIV-Negative Persons

Providing culturally and contextually appropriate messages is essential to help persons at risk avoid contracting HIV infection and to help those who are infected with HIV avoid transmitting the virus. Prevention messages also need to focus on the role of alcohol and drug abuse in HIV risk. Substance abuse (via injection drugs, alcohol, or methamphetamines) can facilitate risky behaviors among persons who might otherwise protect themselves and others from HIV. Preventing substance abuse and increasing access to substance-abuse treatment are examples of effective interventions for reducing HIV transmission.

Integrated Prevention Programs

Federal, state, and local prevention measures are increasingly focused on maximizing public health impact for any given program. One approach to increasing program effectiveness is increasing the development and implementation of integrated HIV-prevention programs. Several integrated programs exist across the nation, combining HIV, sexually transmitted disease (STD), viral hepatitis, mental health, and substance abuse services (25–27). Effective integration requires that program leaders 1) better define program integration goals, 2) identify best practices in the field and ensure that they are disseminated and implemented widely, 3) implement policies and regulations that enhance and support integration at local levels, and 4) evaluate the most cost-effective strategies.

Improved Monitoring of New HIV Infections

Reliable, population-based data are essential to track the HIV epidemic and target prevention measures accurately. For decades, AIDS surveillance has been a cornerstone of national, state, and local efforts to monitor the scope and impact of the HIV epidemic. However, AIDS surveillance data no longer accurately describe the full extent of the epidemic because effective therapies have slowed the progression of the disease. Since 1999, CDC has recommended that states conduct HIV reporting using the same name-based approach currently used for AIDS surveillance nationwide. Currently, 43 states and five territories use confidential, name-based HIV case reporting. Several of the remaining states intend to implement name-based HIV surveillance in 2006. Moreover, in 2006, data from a new national HIV incidence surveillance system will provide the most accurate estimates of new HIV infections. These data, combined with improved surveillance of the patterns and distributions of risk behaviors in the population, will refine the targeting and delivery of HIV-prevention efforts.

New Prevention Technologies

Certain prevention technologies still under development, including preexposure prophylaxis, microbicides, and vaccines, are unlikely to provide full protection against HIV, might offer little or no protection against other STDs such as gonorrhea and chlamydia infections, and will not prevent unwanted pregnancies. Instead, new technologies are more likely to be incorporated into the spectrum of tools for comprehensive approaches to disease prevention. Effective behavior-change programs will still be needed to address possible behavioral disinhibition (i.e., continuing or returning to high-risk behaviors when one feels protected) among persons who receive these interventions. Prevention counseling that addresses informed choice and consent; the HIV-prevention behaviors of abstinence and delay of sexual debut, being monogamous, having fewer sex partners, and using condoms correctly and consistently; and other reproductive health needs (e.g., STD treatment and family planning) must be incorporated alongside these new prevention interventions.

Special Issue of MMWR

HIV/AIDS remains a potentially deadly chronic disease. Prevention of HIV infection requires a continued commitment from persons at risk, persons infected, and society as a whole. Prevention efforts need to keep pace with a changing epidemic. Most importantly, younger generations, who might not remember the deadlier, early days of the epidemic, continually need to receive basic HIV-prevention messages. Twenty-five years after first reporting on AIDS, *MMWR* dedicates this issue to retrospectives on the epidemic, including the changing epidemiology of HIV/AIDS, the public health achievement in reducing perinatal transmission of HIV, and the evolution of measures to prevent HIV/AIDS.

Reported by

K.A. Fenton, R.O. Valdiserri, National Center for HIV/AIDS, Viral Hepatitis, STD and TB Prevention (proposed), CDC.

REFERENCES

1. CDC. *Pneumocystis pneumonia*—Los Angeles. MMWR 1981; 30: 250–52.
2. Glynn MK, Rhodes P. Estimated HIV Prevalence in the United States at the End of 2003 [Abstract T1-B1101]. Presented at the 2005 National HIV Prevention Conference, Atlanta, Georgia; June 14, 2005.
3. CDC. Evolution of HIV Prevention Programs—United States, 1981–2006. MMWR 2006; 55: 597–602.
4. _____. Reduction in Perinatal Transmission of Human Immunodeficiency Virus—United States, 1985–2006. MMWR 2006; 21: 592–97.
5. Dodd RY, Notari EP 4th, Stramer SL. Current Prevalence and Incidence of Infectious Disease Markers and Estimated Window-Period Risk in the American Red Cross Blood Donor Population. Transfusion 2002; 42: 975–79.
6. Anderson JE, Chandra A, Mosher WD. HIV Testing in the United States, 2002. Adv Data 2005; 363: 1–32.

7. MacKellar DA, Valleroy LA, Anderson JE, et al. Recent HIV Testing among Young Men Who Have Sex with Men: Correlates, Contexts, and HIV seroconversion. Sex Transm Dis 2006;33: 183–92.
8. Valdiserri RO. HIV/AIDS in Historical Profile. In: Valdiserri RO, ed. Dawning Answers: How the HIV/AIDS Epidemic Has Helped to Strengthen Public Health. Oxford, England: Oxford University Press; 2003: 3–32.
9. CDC. HIV/AIDS Surveillance Report, 2004. Vol. 16. Atlanta, GA: US Department of Health and Human Services, CDC; 2005. Available at: http://www.cdc.gov/hiv/stats/hasrlink.htm
10. _____. HIV/AIDS among Men Who Have Sex with Men Fact Sheet. Available at http://www.cdc.gov/hiv/pubs/facts/msm.htm.
11. _____. HIV/AIDS Surveillance Report 2003. Vol. 15. Atlanta, GA: US Department of Health and Human Services, CDC; 2004: 1–46.
12. _____. HIV Prevalence, Unrecognized Infection, and HIV Testing among Men Who Have Sex with Men—Five US Cities, June 2004–April 2005. MMWR 2005; 54: 597–601.
13. Dean HD, Steele CB, Satcher AJ, Nakashima AK. HIV/AIDS among Minority Races and Ethnicities in the United States, 1999–2003. J Natl Med Assoc 2005; 97 (7 Suppl): S5–12.
14. CDC. Epidemiology of HIV/AIDS—United States, 1981–2005. MMWR 2006; 55: 589–92.
15. Adapting CDC DEBI list for target audiences is a major issue among CBOs. Translation changes can affect funding. AIDS Alert 2005; 20: 73, 75–8.
16. Amaro H, Blake SM, Morrill AC, et al. HIV Prevention Community Planning: Challenges and Opportunities for Data-Informed Decision-Making. AIDS Behav 2005; 9 (2 Suppl): S9–27.
17. Kates J, Sorian R, Crowley JS, Summers TA. Critical Policy Challenges in the Third Decade of the HIV/AIDS Epidemic. Am J Public Health 2002; 92: 1060–63.
18. Aragon R, Kates J, Hoff T. The AIDS Epidemic at 20 Years: The View from America. Menlo Park, CA: Kaiser Family Foundation; 2001.
19. Valdiserri RO. HIV/AIDS Stigma: an Impediment to Public Health. Am J Public Health 2002; 92: 371–7.
20. Presidential Advisory Council on HIV/AIDS. Achieving an HIV-Free Generation: Recommendations for a New American HIV Strategy. Washington, D.C.: US Department of Health and Human Services; 2006.
21. Marks G, Crepaz N, Senterfitt JW, Janssen RS. Meta-Analysis of High-Risk Sexual Behavior in Persons Aware and Unaware They Are Infected with HIV in the United States: Implications for HIV Prevention Programs. J Acquir Immune Defic Syndr 2005; 39: 446–53.
22. Greenwald JL, Rich CA, Bessega S, Posner MA, Maeda JL, Skolnik PR. Evaluation of the Centers for Disease Control and Prevention's Recommendations Regarding Routine Testing for Human Immunodeficiency Virus by an Inpatient Service: Who Are We Missing? Mayo Clin Proc 2006; 81: 452–8.

23. Chou R, Huffman LH, Fu R, Smits AK, Korthuis PT; US Preventive Services Task Force. Screening for HIV: a Review of the Evidence for the U.S. Preventive Services Task Force. Ann Intern Med 2005; 143: 55–73.

24. CDC. Use of Social Networks to Identify Persons with Undiagnosed HIV Infection—Seven U.S. Cities, October 2003–September 2004. MMWR 2005; 54: 601–5.

25. Gunn RA, Lee MA, Callahan DB, Gonzales P, Murray PJ, Margolis HS. Integrating Hepatitis, STD, and HIV Services into a Drug Rehabilitation Program. Am J Prev Med 2005; 29: 27–33.

26. Gunn RA, Murray PJ, Ackers ML, Hardison WG, Margolis HS. Screening for Chronic Hepatitis B and C Virus Infections in an Urban Sexually Transmitted Disease Clinic: Rationale for Integrating Services. Sex Transm Dis 2001; 28: 166–70.

27. Wilson BC, Moyer L, Schmid G, et al. Hepatitis B Vaccination in Sexually Transmitted Disease (STD) Clinics: A Survey of STD Programs. Sex Transm Dis 2001; 28: 148–52.

Source

Morbidity and Mortality Weekly Reports (MMWR). June 2, 2006: 55(21); 585–589. Accessed online September 2008. http://www.cdc.gov/mmwr/preview/mmwrhtml/mm5521a1.htm?s_cid=mm5521a1_e.

PRESIDENT RONALD REAGAN'S FIRST PUBLIC STATEMENT ON AIDS: SEPTEMBER 17, 1985

The following excerpts are from the transcript of President Ronald Reagan's 32nd news conference. The news conference began at 8:00 p.m. (eastern U.S. time zone) and was broadcast live on television and radio nationwide. These statements record the President's first public mention of AIDS.

The President: Good evening. Please be seated. I have a statement here.

[The President began with a brief statement on economic growth, then responded to questions on a defense topic—the Strategic Defense Initiative. Two questions on federal support for AIDS research followed.]

Question: Mr. President, the nation's best-known AIDS scientist says the time has come now to boost existing research into what he called a minor moonshot program to attack this AIDS epidemic that has struck fear into the Nation's health workers and even its schoolchildren. Would you support a massive government research program against AIDS like the one that President Nixon launched against cancer?

The President: I have been supporting it for more than 4 years now. It's been one of the top priorities with us, and over the last 4 years, and including what we have in the budget for '86, it will amount to over a half a billion dollars that we have provided for research on AIDS in addition to what I'm sure other medical groups are doing. And we have $100 million in the budget this year; it'll be 126 million next year. So, this is a top priority with us. Yes, there's no question about the seriousness of this and the need to find an answer.

Question: If I could follow up, sir. The scientist who talked about this, who does work for the government, is in the National Cancer Institute. He was referring to your program and the increase that you proposed as being not nearly enough at this stage to go forward and really attack the problem.

The President: I think with our budgetary constraints and all, it seems to me that $126 million in a single year for research has got to be something of a vital contribution.

[The news conference continued with Regan fielding questions on an upcoming U.S.–Soviet summit meeting, antisatellite weapons testing, U.S. and Soviet nuclear and space issues, and more on the Strategic Defense Initiative. He was also asked about his personal relationship with Soviet General Secretary Gorbachev and his relationship with Congress, South Africa, and the U.S. Trade Deficit. A question regarding school attendance of children with AIDS followed.]

Question: Mr. President, returning to something that Mike [Mike Putzel, Associated Press] said, if you had younger children, would you send them to a school with a child who had AIDS?

The President: I'm glad I'm not faced with that problem today. And I can well understand the plight of the parents and how they feel about it. I also have compassion, as I think we all do, for the child that has this and doesn't know and can't have it explained to him why somehow he is now an outcast and can no longer associate with his playmates and schoolmates. On the other hand, I can understand the problem with the parents. It is true that some medical sources had said that this cannot be communicated in any way other than the ones we already know and which would not involve a child being in the school. And yet medicine has not come forth unequivocally and said, "This we know for a fact, that it is safe." And until they do, I think we just have to do the best we can with this problem. I can understand both sides of it.

[The news conference continued with questions that again returned to the strategic defense initiative, President Machel of Mozambique, and espionage. It concluded with questions on free and fair trade, with no further mention of HIV/AIDS.]

Source

The full text of the news conference is available at "The President's New Conference. September 17, 1985." The Public Papers of President Ronald W. Reagan. Ronald Reagan Presidential Library. Accessed online October 2008. http://www.reagan.utexas.edu/archives/speeches/1985/91785c.htm

REMARKS AT THE AMERICAN FOUNDATION FOR AIDS RESEARCH AWARDS DINNER, MAY 31, 1987

President Ronald Reagan's First Speech on AIDS. The President spoke at 8:16 p.m. at the Potomac Restaurant. In his opening remarks, he referred to Dr. Mervyn Silverman, president of the American Foundation for AIDS Research; Elizabeth Taylor; and Donald Ross, chairman of the board of New York Life Insurance Co.

The President: Dr. Silverman, Elizabeth, Don Ross, award winners, ladies and gentlemen, I hope Elizabeth won't mind, but some years ago when I was doing a television show, *General Electric Theater*, part of my work required visiting the General Electric plants, 139 of them, and meeting all the employees.

And knowing better than to have a canned speech for them, I would go and suggest that they might ask questions. And every place I went, the first question was "Is Elizabeth Taylor really that pretty?" [Laughter] And being the soul of honesty, I would say, "You bet." [Applause]

But you know, fundraisers always remind me of one of my favorite but most well-worn stories. I've been telling it for years, so if you've heard it, please indulge me. A man had just been elected chairman of his community's annual charity drive. And he went over all the records, and he noticed something about one individual in town, a very wealthy man. And so, he paid a call on him, introduced himself as to what he was doing, and he said, "Our records show that you have never contributed anything to our charity." And the man said, "Well, do your records show that I also have a brother who, as the result of a disabling accident, is permanently disabled and cannot provide for himself? Do your records show that I have an invalid mother and a widowed sister with several small children and no father to support them?" And the chairman, a little abashed and embarrassed, said, "Well, no, our records don't show that." The man said, "Well, I don't give anything to them. Why should I give something to you?" [Laughter]

Well, I do want to thank each of you for giving to the fight against AIDS. And I want to thank the American Foundation for AIDS Research and our award recipients for their contributions, as well. I'm especially pleased a member of the administration is one of tonight's recipients. Dr. [C. Everett] Koop is what every Surgeon General should be. He's an honest man, a good doctor, and an advocate for the public health. I also want to thank other doctors and researchers who aren't here tonight. Those individuals showed genuine courage in the early days of the disease when we didn't know how AIDS was spreading its death. They took personal risks for medical knowledge and for their patients' well-being, and that deserves our gratitude and recognition.

I want to talk tonight about the disease that has brought us all together. It has been talked about, and I'm going to continue. The poet W.H. Auden said that true men of action in our times are not the politicians and statesmen but the scientists. I believe that's especially true when it comes to the AIDS epidemic. Those of us in government can educate our citizens about the dangers. We can encourage safe behavior. We can test to determine how widespread the virus is. We can do any number of things. But only medical science can ever truly defeat AIDS. We've made remarkable progress, as you've heard, already. To think we didn't even know we had a disease until June of 1981, when five cases appeared in California. The AIDS virus itself was discovered in 1984. The blood test became available in 1985. A treatment drug, AZT, has been brought to market in record time, and others are coming. Work on a vaccine is now underway in many laboratories, as you've been told.

In addition to all the private and corporate research underway here at home and around the world, this fiscal year the federal government plans to spend $317 million on AIDS research and $766 million overall. Next year we intend to spend 30 percent more on research: $413 million out of $1 billion overall. Spending on AIDS has been one of the fastest growing parts of the budget, and, ladies and gentlemen, it deserves to be. We're also tearing down the regulatory barriers so as to move AIDS from the pharmaceutical laboratory to the marketplace as quickly as possible. It makes no sense, and in fact it's cruel, to keep the hope of new drugs from dying patients. And I don't blame those who are out marching and protesting to get AIDS drugs released before [. . .] the T's were crossed and the I's were dotted. I sympathize with them, and we'll supply help and hope as quickly as we can.

Science is clearly capable of breathtaking advances, but it's not capable of miracles. Because of AIDS long incubation period, it'll take years to know if a vaccine works. These tests require time, and this is a problem money cannot overcome. We will not have a vaccine on the market until the mid- to late 1990's, at best. Since we don't have a cure for the disease and we don't have a vaccine against it, the question is how do we deal with it in the meantime. How do we protect the citizens of this nation, and where do we start? For one thing, it's absolutely essential that the American people understand the nature and the extent of the AIDS problem. And it's important that federal and state governments do the same.

I recently announced my intention to create a national commission on AIDS because of the consequences of this disease on our society. We need some comprehensive answers. What can we do to defend Americans not infected with the virus? How can we best care for those who are ill and dying? How do we deal with a disease that may swamp our health care system? The commission will help crystallize America's best ideas on how to deal with the AIDS crisis. We know some things already: the cold statistics. But I'm not going to read you gruesome facts on how many thousands have died or most certainly will die. I'm not going to break down the numbers and categories of those we've lost, because I don't want Americans to think AIDS simply affects only certain groups. AIDS affects all of us.

What our citizens must know is this: America faces a disease that is fatal and spreading. And this calls for urgency, not panic. It calls for compassion, not blame. And it calls for understanding, not ignorance. It's also important that America not reject those who have the disease, but care for them with dignity and kindness. Final judgment is up to God; our part is to ease the suffering and to find a cure. This is a battle against disease, not against our fellow Americans. We mustn't allow those with the AIDS virus to suffer discrimination. I agree with Secretary of Education Bennett: We must firmly oppose discrimination against those who have AIDS. We must prevent the persecution, through ignorance or malice, of our fellow citizens.

As dangerous and deadly as AIDS is, many of the fears surrounding it are unfounded. These fears are based on ignorance. I was told of a newspaper photo of a baby in a hospital crib with a sign that said, "AIDS—Do Not Touch." Fortunately, that photo was taken several years ago, and we now know there's no basis for this kind of fear. But similar incidents are still happening elsewhere in this country. I read of one man with AIDS who returned to work to find anonymous notes on his desk with such messages as, "Don't use our water fountain." I was told of a situation in Florida where 3 young brothers—ages 10, 9, and 7—were all hemophiliacs carrying the AIDS virus. The pastor asked the entire family not to come back to their church. Ladies and gentlemen, this is old-fashioned fear, and it has no place in the "home of the brave."

The Public Health Service has stated that there's no medical reason for barring a person with the virus from any routine school or work activity. There's no reason for those who carry the AIDS virus to wear a scarlet A. AIDS is not a casually contagious disease. We're still learning about how AIDS is transmitted, but experts tell us you don't get it from telephones or swimming pools or drinking fountains. You don't get it from shaking hands or sitting on a bus or anywhere else, for that matter. And most important, you don't get AIDS by donating blood. Education is critical to clearing up the fears. Education is also crucial to stopping the transmission of the disease. Since we don't yet have a cure or a vaccine, the only thing that can halt the spread of AIDS right now is a change in the behavior of those Americans who are at risk.

As I've said before, the federal role is to provide scientific, factual information. Corporations can help get the information out, so can community and religious groups, and of course so can the schools, with guidance from the parents and with the commitment, I hope, that AIDS education or any aspect of sex education will not be value-neutral. A dean of St. Paul's Cathedral in London once said: "The aim of education is the knowledge not of facts, but of values." Well, that's not too far off. Education is knowing how to adapt, to grow, to understand ourselves and the world around us. And values are how we guide ourselves through the decisions of life. How we behave sexually is one of those decisions. As Surgeon General Koop has pointed out, if children are taught their own worth, we can expect them to treat themselves and others with greater respect. And wherever you have self-respect and mutual respect, you don't have drug abuse and sexual promiscuity, which of course are the two major causes of AIDS. Nancy, too, has found from her work that self-esteem is the best defense against drug abuse.

Now, we know there will be those who will go right ahead. So, yes, after there is a moral base, then you can discuss preventives and other scientific measures. And there's another aspect of teaching values that needs to be mentioned here. As individuals, we have a moral obligation not to endanger others, and that can mean endangering others with a gun, with a car, or with a virus. If a person has reason to believe that he or she may be a carrier, that person has a moral duty to be tested for AIDS; human decency requires it. And the reason is very simple: Innocent people are being infected by this virus, and some of them are going to acquire AIDS and die.

Let me tell you a story about innocent, unknowing people. A doctor in a rural county in Kentucky treated a woman who caught the AIDS virus from her husband, who was an IV-drug user. They later got divorced, neither knowing that they were infected. They remarried other people, and now one of them has already transmitted the disease to her new husband. Just as most individuals don't know they carry the virus, no one knows to what extent the virus has infected our entire society. AIDS is surreptitiously spreading throughout our population, and yet we have no accurate measure of its scope. It's time we knew exactly what we were facing, and that's why I support some routine testing.

I've asked the Department of Health and Human Services to determine as soon as possible the extent to which the AIDS virus has penetrated our society and to predict its future dimensions. I've also asked HHS to add the AIDS virus to the list of contagious diseases for which immigrants and aliens seeking permanent residence in the United States can be denied entry.

Audience members: [Booing]

The President: They are presently denied entry for other contagious diseases. I've asked the Department of Justice to plan for testing all federal prisoners, as looking into ways to protect uninfected inmates and their families. In addition, I've asked for a review of other federal responsibilities, such as veterans' hospitals, to see if testing might be appropriate in those areas. This is in addition to the testing already underway in our military and foreign service.

Audience members: No! No!

The President: Now let me turn to what the states can do. Some are already at work. While recognizing the individual's choice, I encourage states to offer routine testing for those who seek marriage licenses and for those who visit sexually transmitted disease or drug abuse clinics. And I encourage states to require routine testing in state and local prisons. Not only will testing give us more information on which to make decisions, but in the case of marriage licenses, it might prevent at least some babies from being born with AIDS. And anyone who knows how viciously AIDS attacks the body cannot object to this humane consideration. I should think that everyone getting married would want to be tested.

You know, it's been said that when the night is darkest, we see the stars. And there have been some shining moments throughout this horrible AIDS epidemic. I'm talking about all those volunteers across the country who've ministered to the sick and the helpless. For example, last year about 450 volunteers from the Shanti Project provided 130,000 hours of emotional and practical support for 87 percent of San Francisco's AIDS patients. That kind of compassion has been duplicated all over the country, and it symbolizes the best tradition of caring. And I encourage Americans to follow that example and volunteer to help their fellow citizens who have AIDS.

In closing, let me read to you something I saw in the paper that also embodies the American spirit. It's something that a young man with AIDS recently said. He said: "While I do accept death, I think the fight for life is important, and I'm going to fight the disease with every breath I have." Ladies and gentlemen, so must we. Thank you.

Source

"Remarks at the American Foundation for AIDS Research Awards Dinner, May 31, 1987." *The Public Papers of President Ronald W. Reagan.* Ronald Reagan Presidential Library. Accessed online December 2008. http://www.reagan.utexas.edu/archives/speeches/1987/053187a.htm.

Rumors, Myths, and Hoaxes

The CDC responds to several widely circulated items of misinformation.

I got an e-mail warning that a man, who was believed to be HIV-positive, was recently caught placing blood in the ketchup dispenser at a fast food restaurant. Because of the risk of HIV transmission, the e-mail recommended that only individually wrapped packets of ketchup be used. Is there a risk of contracting HIV from ketchup?

No incidents of ketchup dispensers being contaminated with HIV-infected blood have been reported to CDC. Furthermore, CDC has no reports of HIV infection resulting from eating food, including condiments.

HIV is not an airborne or food-borne virus, and it does not live long outside the body. Even if small amounts of HIV-infected blood were consumed, stomach acid would destroy the virus. Therefore, there is no risk of contracting HIV from eating ketchup.

HIV is most commonly transmitted through specific sexual behaviors (anal, vaginal, or oral sex) or needle sharing with an infected person. An HIV-infected woman can pass the virus to her baby before or during childbirth or after birth through breastfeeding. Although the risk is extremely low in the United Stats, it is also possible to acquire HIV through transfusions of infected blood or blood products.

Did a Texas child die of a heroin overdose after being stuck by a used needle found on a playground?

This story was investigated and found to be a hoax. To become overdosed on a drug from a used needle and syringe, a person would have to have a large amount of the drug injected directly into their body. A needle stick injury such as that mentioned in the story would not lead to a large enough injection to cause a drug overdose. In addition, drug users would leave very little drug material in a discarded syringe after they have injected. If such an incident were to happen, there would likely be concerns about possible blood borne infections, such as human immunodeficiency virus and hepatitis B or C. The risk of these infections from an improperly disposed of needle, such as that described in the story, are extremely low.

Can HIV be transmitted through contact with unused feminine (sanitary) pads?

HIV cannot be transmitted through the use of new, unused feminine pads. The human immunodeficiency virus, or HIV, is a virus that is passed from one person to another through blood-to-blood and sexual contact with someone who is infected with HIV. In addition, infected pregnant women can pass HIV to their babies during pregnancy or delivery, as well as through breast feeding. Although some people have been concerned that HIV might be transmitted in other ways, such as through air, water, insects, or common objects, no scientific evidence supports this. Even though no one has gotten HIV from touching used feminine pads, used pads should be wrapped and properly disposed of so no one comes in contact with blood.

Is a weekly world news story that claims CDC has discovered a mutated version of HIV that is transmitted through the air true?

This story is **not** true. It is unfortunate that such stories, which may frighten the public, are being circulated on the Internet.

Human immunodeficiency virus (HIV), the virus that causes AIDS, is spread by sexual contact (anal, vaginal, or oral) or by sharing needles and/or syringes with someone who is infected with HIV.

Babies born to HIV-infected women may become infected before or during birth or through breast feeding.

Many scientific studies have been done to look at all the possible ways that HIV is transmitted. These studies have not shown HIV to be transmitted through air, water, insects, or casual contact.

I have read stories on the Internet about people getting stuck by needles in phone booth coin returns, movie theater seats, gas pump handles, and other places. One story said that CDC reported similar incidents about improperly discarded needles and syringes. Are these stories true?

CDC has received inquiries about a variety of reports or warnings about used needles left by HIV-infected injection drug users in coin return slots of pay phones, the underside of gas pump handles, and on movie theater seats. These reports and warnings have been circulated on the Internet and by e-mail and fax. Some reports have falsely indicated that CDC "confirmed" the presence of HIV in the needles. CDC has not tested such needles nor has CDC confirmed the presence or absence of HIV in any sample related to these rumors. The majority of these reports and warnings appear to have no foundation in fact.

CDC was informed of one incident in Virginia of a needle stick from a small-gauge needle (believed to be an insulin needle) in a coin return slot of a pay phone. The incident was investigated by the local police department. Several days later, after a report of this police action appeared in the local newspaper, a needle was found in a vending machine but did not cause a needle-stick injury.

Discarded needles are sometimes found in the community outside of health care settings. These needles are believed to have been discarded by persons who use insulin or are injection drug users. Occasionally the "public" and certain groups of workers (e.g., sanitation workers or housekeeping staff) may sustain needle-stick injuries involving inappropriately discarded needles. Needle-stick injuries can transfer blood and blood-borne pathogens (e.g., hepatitis B, hepatitis C, and HIV), but the risk of transmission from discarded needles is extremely low.

CDC does not recommend testing discarded needles to assess the presence or absence of infectious agents in the needles. Management of exposed persons should be done on a case-by-case evaluation of (1) the risk of a blood-borne pathogen infection in the source and (2) the nature of the injury. Anyone who is injured from a needle stick in a community setting should contact their physician or go to an emergency room as soon as possible. The health care professional should then report the injury to the local or state health department. CDC is not aware of any cases where HIV has been transmitted by a needle-stick injury outside a health care setting.

Source

"Rumors, Myths, and Hoaxes." 2007. Centers for Disease Control and Prevention (CDC). March 8. CDC Web site. Retrieved online November 2008. HTTP://WWW.CDC.GOV/HIV/RESOURCES/QA/HOAX1.HTM.

HOW SAFE IS THE BLOOD SUPPLY IN THE UNITED STATES?

The CDC's statement addressing concerns regarding the U.S. blood supply and HIV.

The U.S. blood supply is among the safest in the world. Nearly all people infected with HIV through blood transfusions received those transfusions before 1985, the year HIV testing began for all donated blood.

The Public Health Service has recommended an approach to blood safety in the United States that includes stringent donor selection practices and the use of screening tests. U.S. blood donations have been screened for antibodies to HIV-1 since March 1985 and HIV-2 since June 1992. The p24 Antigen test was added in 1996. Blood and blood products that test positive for HIV are safely discarded and are not used for transfusions.

Tests Performed on Each Unit of Donated Blood

Disease	Test	Year Implemented
HIV/AIDS	HIV/AIDS HIV- I Antibody test	1985
	HIV-1/2 Antibody test	1992
	HIV-I p24 Antigen test	1996
HIV/AIDS and Hepatitis C	Nucleic Acid Test (NAT)	1999
Hepatitis C	Hepatitis C Anti-HCV	1990
Hepatitis B	Hepatitis B Surface Antigen test	1971
	Hepatitis B Core Antibody	1987
Hepatitis	Hepatitis ALT	1986
Syphilis	Syphilis Serologic test	1948
Human T-cell Lymphotropic Virus (HTLV)	HTLV-I Antibody	1989
	HTLV-I/II Antibody	1998

Source: American Red Cross.

The improvement of processing methods for blood products also has reduced the number of infections resulting from the use of these products.

Currently, the risk of infection with HIV in the United States through receiving a blood transfusion or blood products is extremely low and has become progressively lower, even in geographic areas with high HIV prevalence rates.

This list is subject to change as new blood safety opportunities and requirements emerge. Additional tests may be performed to meet special patient needs.

Date: October 20, 2006

Source

Centers for Disease Control and Prevention (CDC). Accessed online December 2008. http://www.cdc.gov/hiv/resources/qa/qa15.htm.

DECIDING IF AND WHEN TO BE TESTED

The CDC's guidance on being tested for HIV, the virus that causes AIDS.

Should I Get Tested?

The following are behaviors that increase your chances of getting HIV. If you answer yes to any of them, you should definitely get an HIV test. If you continue with any of these behaviors, you should be tested every year. Talk to a health care provider about an HIV testing schedule that is right for you.

- Have you injected drugs or steroids or shared equipment (such as needles, syringes, works) with others?
- Have you had unprotected vaginal, anal, or oral sex with men who have sex with men, multiple partners, or anonymous partners?
- Have you exchanged sex for drugs or money?
- Have you been diagnosed with or treated for hepatitis, tuberculosis (TB), or a sexually transmitted disease (STD), like syphilis?
- Have you had unprotected sex with someone who could answer yes to any of the above questions?

If you have had sex with someone whose history of sex partners and/or drug use is unknown to you or if you or your partner has had many sex partners, then you have more of a chance of being infected with HIV. Both you and your new partner should get tested for HIV, and learn the results, before having sex for the first time.

For women who plan to become pregnant, testing is even more important. If a woman is infected with HIV, medical care and certain drugs given during pregnancy can lower the chance of passing HIV to her baby. All women who are pregnant should be tested during each pregnancy.

How Long after a Possible Exposure Should I Wait to Get Tested for HIV?

Most HIV tests are antibody tests that measure the antibodies your body makes against HIV. It can take some time for the immune system to produce enough antibodies for the antibody test to detect, and this time period can vary from person to person. This time period is commonly referred to as the "window period." Most people will develop detectable antibodies within 2 to 8 weeks (the average is 25 days). Even so, there is a chance that some individuals will take longer to develop detectable antibodies. Therefore, if the initial negative HIV test was conducted within the first 3 months after possible exposure, repeat testing should be considered >3 months after the exposure occurred to account for the possibility of a false-negative result. Ninety-seven percent of persons will develop antibodies in the first 3 months following the time of their infection. In very rare cases, it can take up to 6 months to develop antibodies to HIV.

Another type of test is an RNA test, which detects the HIV virus directly. The time between HIV infection and RNA detection is 9–11 days. These tests, which are more costly and used less often than antibody tests, are used in some parts of the United States.

For information on HIV testing, you can talk to your health care provider or you can find the location of the HIV testing site nearest to you by visiting the National HIV Testing Resources Web site at http://www.hivtest.org or call CDC-INFO 24 Hours/Day at 1-800-CDC-INFO (232-4636), 1-888-232-6348 (TTY), in English, en Español. Both of these resources are confidential.

If you would like more information or have personal concerns, call CDC-INFO 24 Hours/Day at 1-800-CDC-INFO (232-4636), 1-888-232-6348 (TTY), in English, en Español.

Source

Centers for Disease Control and Prevention (CDC). 2007. "Deciding If and When to Be Tested." CDC Web site. Accessed online December 2008. http://www.cdc.gov/hiv/topics/testing/resources/qa/be_tested.htm.

Directory of Organizations

U.S. FEDERAL ORGANIZATIONS

Department of Health and Human Services (DHHS)

http://www.hhs.gov

In the United States, the Department of Health and Human Services (DHHS) "is the United States government's principal agency for protecting the health of all Americans and providing essential human services, especially for those who are least able to help themselves." The DHHS includes more than 300 programs, including several agencies and offices that have responsibilities for responding to the HIV/AIDS pandemic. Some of these programs are listed below.

Centers for Disease Control and Prevention (CDC)

http://www.cdc.gov

The Centers for Disease Control and Prevention (CDC) is an agency of the Department of Health and Human Services (DHHS). The CDC conducts and supports public health activities in the United States. The CDC's mission is "to promote health and quality of life by preventing and controlling disease, injury, and disability." Epidemiologists from the CDC took the lead in investigating the early cases of AIDS, and the CDC continues to track prevalence and provide information on HIV and AIDS.

Food and Drug Administration (FDA)

http://www.fda.gov

The Food and Drug Administration (FDA) is an agency of the DHHS. The FDA is responsible for "protecting the public health by assuring the safety, efficacy, and security of human and veterinary drugs, biological products, medical devices, [the] nation's food supply, cosmetics, and products that emit radiation.

The FDA is also responsible for advancing the public health by helping to speed innovations that make medicines and foods more effective, safer, and more affordable; and helping the public get the accurate, science-based information they need to use medicines and foods to improve their health." The safety of the nation's blood supply is part of the FDA's responsibility.

National Institutes of Health (NIH)

http://www.nih.gov

The National Institutes of Health (NIH), comprising 27 Institutes and Centers, is an agency of the DHHS. The NIH conducts medical research on disease cause, treatment, and cure. It also invests billions of dollars annually in financial support of medical research in the U.S. and around the world. Researchers at the NIH have been active in researching AIDS from the early days of the crisis. HIV/AIDS is a specific mission area of one of these institutes, specifically the National Institute of Allergy and Infectious Diseases. The scientific, budgetary, legislative, and policy elements of the NIH research program are handled through the Office of AIDS Research (http://www.oar.nih.gov/).

Office of Public Health and Science (OPHS)

http://www.hhs.gov/ophs/index.html

The Secretary of the Department of Health and Human Services oversees the Office of Public Health and Science (OPHS). The OPHS comprises 12 core public health offices and the U.S. Public Health Service. The Office of the Surgeon General (OSG) and the Office of HIV/AIDS Policy (OHAP) are two of these core offices.

Office of the Surgeon General (OSG)

http://www.surgeongeneral.gov

The Surgeon General oversees this office. The Surgeon General is a physician who "serves as America's chief health educator by providing Americans the best scientific information available on how to improve their health and reduce the risk of illness and injury." This means that "the role of the Surgeon General is to protect and advance the health of the nation." The Surgeon General has informed HIV/AIDS educational efforts throughout the pandemic.

Office of HIV/AIDS Policy (OHAP)

http://www.hhs.gov/ophs/ohap

The Office of HIV/AIDS Policy (OHAP) advises federal health officials on "the appropriate and timely implementation and development of HIV/AIDS policy; the establishment of priorities; and the implementation of HIV/AIDS programs, activities, and initiatives across other HHS health agencies." It oversees the "National HIV Testing Mobilization Campaign" (http://www.aids.gov/takecontrol/) that promotes HIV testing as well as the AIDS.gov (http://aids.gov/) informational portal that provides access to a wealth of U.S. HIV/AIDS information.

INTERNATIONAL ORGANIZATIONS

Tracking data on HIV/AIDS around the world is a daunting and difficult task. Two organizations that have primarily undertaken that effort, and work to fight the pandemic, are the World Health Organization (WHO) and the Joint United Nations Programme on HIV/AIDS (UNAIDS).

World Health Organization (WHO)

http://www.who.int/en

The WHO is the directing and coordinating authority for health within the United Nations system. It is responsible for providing leadership on global health matters, shaping the health research agenda, setting norms and standards, articulating evidence-based policy options, providing technical support to countries and monitoring and assessing health trends. The WHO serves as a data-collection clearinghouse for compilation and analysis on HIV/AIDS data much like the Centers for Disease Control and Prevention (CDC) does for the United States.

Joint United Nations Programme on HIV/AIDS (UNAIDS)

http://www.unaids.org/en

UNAIDS brings together the efforts and resources of ten United Nations system organizations to help prevent new HIV infections, care for people living with HIV, and mitigate the impact of the pandemic globally. The organization works in more than 80 countries worldwide. Cosponsors include the United Nations High Commissioner for Refugees (UNHCR), United Nations Children's Fund (UNICEF), World Food Programme (WFP), United Nations Development Programme (UNDP), United Nations Population Fund (UNFPA), United Nations Office on Drugs and Crime (UNODC), International Labour Organization (ILO), United Nations Educational, Scientific and Cultural Organization (UNESCO), World Health Organization (WHO), and the World Bank.

GLOSSARY

Acquired Immunodeficiency Syndrome (AIDS) A disease of the body's immune system caused by the human immunodeficiency virus (HIV). AIDS is characterized by the death of CD4 cells (an important part of the body's immune system), which leaves the body vulnerable to life-threatening conditions such as infections and cancers.

Antibody A protein produced by the body's immune system that recognizes and fights infectious organisms and other foreign substances that enter the body. Each antibody is specific to a particular piece of an infectious organism or other foreign substance.

Antiretroviral (ARV) A medication that interferes with the ability of a retrovirus (such as HIV) to make more copies of itself.

Antiretroviral Therapy (ART) Treatment with drugs that inhibit the ability of retroviruses (such as HIV) to multiply in the body. The antiretroviral therapy recommended for HIV infection is referred to as highly active antiretroviral therapy (HAART).

Asymptomatic Having no obvious signs or symptoms of disease.

Baseline An initial measurement (for example, CD4 count or viral load) made before starting treatment or therapy for a disease or condition.

Co-Infection Infection with more than one virus, bacterium, or other microorganism at a given time. For example, an HIV-infected individual may be co-infected with hepatitis C virus (HCV) or tuberculosis (TB).

Effectiveness The measure of the success of a treatment for a particular disease or condition.

Efficacy The ability of a treatment to produce the desired effect on the disease or condition being treated.

Endemic A term that refers to diseases associated with particular geographic regions or populations.

Highly Active Antiretroviral Therapy (HAART) The name given to treatment regimens that aggressively suppress HIV replication and progression of HIV disease.

Human Immunodeficiency Virus (HIV) The virus that causes Acquired Immunodeficiency Syndrome (AIDS). HIV is in the retrovirus family, and two types have been identified: HIV-1 and HIV-2. HIV-1 is responsible for most HIV infections throughout the world, while HIV-2 is found primarily in West Africa.

Immune System The collection of cells and organs whose role is to protect the body from foreign invaders.

Immunodeficiency Inability to produce normal amounts of antibodies, immune cells, or both.

Incidence The rate of occurrence of new cases of a particular disease in a given population. Often reported as number of cases per 100,000 people.

Kaposi's Sarcoma (KS) A type of cancer caused by an overgrowth of blood vessels, which causes pink or purple spots or small bumps on the skin.

Lesion An area of the body where tissue is abnormal, such as an infected patch or sore on the skin.

Macrophage A type of disease-fighting white blood cell that destroys foreign invaders and stimulates other immune system cells to fight infection.

Neonatal The time period from birth through the first four weeks after birth.

Opportunistic Infections (OIs) Illnesses caused by various organisms that occur in people with weakened immune systems, including people with HIV/AIDS.

Postnatal The time period following birth (refers to the newborn).

Prenatal Period of time spanning conception to the beginning of labor.

Remission The period during which symptoms of a disease diminish or disappear.

Viral Load (VL) The amount of HIV RNA in a blood sample, reported as number of HIV RNA copies per mL of blood plasma. The VL provides information about the number of cells infected with HIV and is an important indicator of HIV progression and how well treatment is working.

REFERENCE

AIDSinfo. 2005. *Glossary of HIV/AIDS Related Terms*. U.S. DHHS: Rockville, MD. Accessed online December 2008. http://www.aidsinfo.nih.gov/ContentFiles/GlossaryHIVrelatedTerms.pdf.

FURTHER READING

This selected bibliography provides a range of materials complementing the content of this volume and representing the range of current scholarship and perspectives on HIV/AIDS. Because the extensive body of literature on HIV/AIDS is constantly evolving, it is not offered as an exhaustive directory of available materials. Indeed, it is doubtful that such a list would even be possible, given the plethora of available materials.

HISTORY OF HIV/AIDS

Engel, Jonathan. 2006. *The Epidemic: A Global History of AIDS*. New York: Smithsonian Books/Collins.

Grmek, M.D. 1989. *History of AIDS: Emergence and Origins of a Modern Pandemic*. Princeton, NJ: Princeton University Press.

Shilts, Randy. 1987. *And the Band Played On: Politics, People, and the AIDS Epidemic*. New York: St. Martin's Press.

HIV/AIDS DENIERS/DISSENTERS

Bauer, Henry H. 2007. *The Origin, Persistence, and Failings of HIV/AIDS Theory*. Jefferson, NC: McFarland and Company.

Culshaw, Rebecca. 2007. *Science Sold Out: Does HIV Really Cause AIDS?* Berkeley: CA: North Atlantic Books.

Duesberg, Peter H. 1997. *Inventing the AIDS Virus*. Washington, D.C.: Regnery.

Duesberg, Peter H., and John Yiamouyiannis. 1995. *AIDS: The Good News Is HIV Doesn't Cause It*. Delaware, OH: Health Action Press.

Maggiore, Christine. 2006. *What if Everything You Thought you Knew about AIDS Was Wrong?* Studio City, CA: American Foundation for AIDS Alternatives.

INTERNATIONAL

Barnett, Tony and Alan Whiteside. 2006. *AIDS in the Twenty-First Century: Disease and Globalization*, 2nd ed. New York: Palgrave Macmillan.

Baylies, Corolyn and Janet Burja with the Gender and AIDS Group. 2000. *AIDS, Sexuality, and Gender in Africa: Strategies and Struggles in Tanzania and Zambia*. New York/London: Routledge.

Beyrer, Chris. 1998. *War in the Blood: Sex, Politics, and AIDS in Southeast Asia*. London: Zed Books.

Eldis–HIV/AIDS Topic area Focuses on international development policy, practice and research http://www.eldis.org/go/topics/resource-guides/hiv-and-aids

Epstein, Helen. 2008. *The Invisible Cure: Why We Are Losing the Fight Against AIDS in Africa*. New York: Picador.

Feldman, Douglas A. 2008. *AIDS, Culture, and Africa*. Gainesville, FL: University Press of Florida.

Irwin, Alexander, Joyce Millen, and Dorothy Fallows. 2003. *Global AIDS: Myths and Facts-Tools for Fighting the AIDS Pandemic*. Cambridge, MA: South End Press.

Kalipeni, Ezekiel, Susan Craddock, Joseph R. Oppong, and Jayati Ghosh, eds. 2003. *HIV and AIDS in Africa: Beyond Epidemiology*. Oxford: Blackwell.

Nolen, Stephanie. 2008. *28: Stories of AIDS in Africa*. New York: Walker and Company.

Pan American Health Organization AIDS and STI Information http://devserver.paho.org/hq/index.php?option=com_content&task=view&id=273&Itemid=370

Rodlach, Alexander. 2006. *Witches, Westerners, and HIV: AIDS and Cultures of Blame in Africa*. Walnut Creek, CA: Left Coast Press.

Sen, Amartya. 2008. *AIDS Sutra: Untold Stories from India*. New York: Anchor.

UNAIDS The Joint United Nations Programme on HIV/AIDS, cosponsored by a variety of international organizations http://www.unaids.org/en/.

JOURNALS (HIV/AIDS SPECIFIC OR RELATED, ACADEMIC)

AIDS
AIDS and Behavior
AIDS Care
AIDS Clinical Care
AIDS Education and Prevention
AIDS Patient Care

AIDS Reader
AIDS Research and Human Retroviruses
AIDS Reviews
Future HIV Therapy
HIV Medicine
International Journal of STD and AIDS
Journal of Acquired Immune Deficiency Syndromes (JAIDS)
Journal of the International AIDS Society
Journal of Sex Research
Morbidity & Mortality Weekly Report (MMWR)
Retrovirology
Sexually Transmitted Diseases
Sexually Transmitted Infections
Journal Watch for HIV/AIDS.
Summaries of medical literature.
http://aids-clinical-care.jwatch.org/.

LIVING WITH HIV/AIDS/PERSONAL EXPERIENCES

A&U Magazine: http://www.aumag.org/.
Bayer, Ronald and Gerald M. Oppenheimer. 2000. *AIDS Doctors: Voices from the Epidemic: An Oral History*. New York: Oxford University Press.
Being Alive Support Organization: http://www.beingalivela.org/
Draper, Nancy D. 2004. *A Burden of Silence: My Mother's Battle with AIDS*. Bloomington, IN: AuthorHouse.
HIVPlus Magazine: http://www.hivplus.com/.
HIV Positive! Magazine: http://www.hivpositivemagazine.com/.
Hoffman, Amy. 1997. *Hospital Time*. Durham, NC: Duke University Press.
Klitzman, Robert. 1997. *Being Positive: The Lives of Men and Women with HIV*. Chicago: Ivan R. Dee.
Klitzman, Robert, and Ronald Bayer. 2003. *Mortal Secrets: Truth and Lies in the Age of AIDS*. Baltimore, MD: Johns Hopkins University Press.
Mayo-Smith, Ian, and Catherine Wyatt-Morley. 2005. *Positive People*. Sterling, VA: Kumarian Press.
Monette, Paul. 1998. *Borrowed Time: An AIDS Memoir*. Fort Washington, PA: Harvest Books.
mPowrPlus Magazine: http://www.mpowrplus.com/.
Positively Aware. The Journal of the Test Positive Aware Network: http://www.tpan.com/.
POSORNOT: Quiz and information about assumption regarding who is HIV+: http://www.posornot.com/.
POZ Magazine. http://www.poz.com/
Weitz, Rose. 1991. *Life With AIDS*. Piscataway, NJ: Rutgers.

Whetten-Goldstein, Kathryn and Trang Quyen Nguyen. 2003. *You're the First One I've Told: New Faces of HIV in the South.* New Brunswick, NJ: Rutgers University Press.

Wooten, Jim. 2005. *We Are All the Same: A Story of a Boy's Courage and a Mother's Love.* New York: Penguin.

Wyatt-Morley, Catherine. 1997. *AIDS Memoir: Journal of an HIV-Positive Mother.* Sterling, VA: Kumarian Press.

MEDICAL ASPECTS

Food and Drug Administration (FDA): http://www.fda.gov/.

National Institutes of Health (NIH): http://www.nih.gov/.

OVERVIEWS/GENERAL INFORMATION

AIDS clock: http://www.poz.ca/aids_clock.htm.

AIDS Education and Training Centers: National Resource Center: http://www.aids-ed.org/.

AIDS Education Global Information System (AEGIS): The world's largest free-access virtual AIDS library: http://www.aegis.com/.

AIDS InfoNet: This project of the New Mexico AIDS Education and Training Center at the University of New Mexico Health Sciences Center provides outreach information in several languages: http://www.aidsinfonet.org/.

AVERTing HIV and AIDS (AVERT): Informative Web site of an international AIDS charity headquartered in the United Kingdom: http://www.avert.org/.

The Body: Informative Web site providing a range of HIV/AIDS information: http://www.thebody.com/.

Fan, Hung Y., Ross F. Conner, and Luis P. Villareal. 2007. *AIDS: Science and Society,* 5th ed. Boston: Jones and Bartlett.

HIV/AIDS Search Engine: Search engine specifically for information on HIV and AIDS: http://www.hivaidssearch.com/.

Kaiser Family Foundation: http://www.kff.org/hivaids/index.cfm.

Stine, Gerald. 2008. *AIDS Update 2008.* Boston: McGraw Hill. (This is the 17th edition of this annual series. A more recent version may be available.)

Whiteside, Alan. 2008. *HIV/AIDS: A Very Short Introduction.* New York: Oxford University Press.

POLICY ISSUES

ACT-UP: The influential social justice activist movement: www.actupny.org.

AIDS Action: National HIV/AIDS advocacy organization: http://www.aidsaction.org/.

Balin, Jane. 1999. *A Neighborhood Divided: Community Resistance to an AIDS Care Facility*. Ithaca: Cornell University Press.

Behrman, Greg. 2004. *The Invisible People: How the United States Slept Through the Global AIDS Pandemic, the Greatest Humanitarian Disaster of Our Time*. New York: Free Press.

Boehmer, Ulrike. 2000. *The Personal and the Political: Women's Activism in Response to the Breast Cancer and AIDS Epidemic*. Albany, NY: State University of New York.

Cochrane, Michelle. 2003. *When AIDS Began: San Francisco and the Making of an Epidemic*. New York: Routledge.

Epstein, Steven. 1996. *Impure Science: AIDS, Activism, and the Politics of Knowledge*. Berkeley/Los Angeles: University of California Press.

Farmer, Paul. 1992. *AIDS and Accusations: Haiti and the Geography of Blame*. Berkeley: University of California.

_____. 1999. *Infections and Inequalities: The Modern Plagues*. Berkeley: University of California.

Gay Men's Health Crisis (GMHC): Advocacy organization since 1982: http://www.gmhc.org/.

Office of HIV/AIDS Policy (OHAP): http://www.hhs.gov/ophs/ohap/.

Public Health Watch. 2006. *HIV/AIDS Policy in the United States: Monitoring the UNGASS Declaration of Commitment on HIV/AIDS*. New York: Open Society Institute. Available at: http://www.soros.org/initiatives/health/focus/phw/articles_publications/publications/hivaids_20060523.

Singer, Merrill. 1998. *The Political Economy of AIDS*. Amityville, NY: Baywood Publishing.

Siplon, Patricia D. 2002. *AIDS and the Policy Struggle in the United States*. Washington, D.C.: Georgetown University.

Theodoulou, Stella Z. 1996. *AIDS and the Politics and Policy of Disease*. Upper Saddle River, NJ: Prentice Hall.

POPULAR CULTURE, MEDIA, AND THE ARTS

Altman, Dennis. 1986. *AIDS in the Mind of America*. New York: Anchor.

Fee, Elizabeth and Daniel M. Fox. 1992. *AIDS: The Making of a Chronic Disease*. Berkeley/Los Angeles: University of California Press. 1992.

Kinsella, James. 1989. *Covering the Plague: AIDS and the American Media*. New Brunswick, NJ: Rutgers University Press.

Klusacek, Alan, and Ken Morrison, eds. 1992. *A Leap in the Dark: AIDS, Art, and Contemporary Cultures*. Montréal: Véhicule Press.

Miller, James. 1992. *Fluid Exchanges: Artists and Critics in the AIDS Crisis*. Toronto: University of Toronto Press.

Watney, Simon. 1987. *Policing Desire: Pornography, AIDS, and the Media*. Minneapolis: University of Minnesota Press.

PREVALENCE DATA

Centers for Disease Control and Prevention (CDC): http://www.cdc.gov/
State and Local HIV/AIDS Surveillance: http://www.cdc.gov/hiv/topics/surveillance/
    resources/reports/2006report/webaddress.htm
World Health Organization (WHO) HIV/AIDS Information: http://www.who.int/
    topics/hiv_aids/en/.

PUBLIC HEALTH, PLAGUES IN HISTORY, AND EMERGING DISEASES

Doka, Kenneth J. 1997. *AIDS, Fear, and Society: Challenging the Dreaded Disease.* Bristol, PA: Taylor & Francis.

Garrett, Laurie. 2002. *Betrayal of Trust: The Collapse of Global Public Health.*

_____. 1995. *The Coming Plague: Newly Emerging Diseases in a World out of Balance.* New York: Penguin.

Karlen, Arno. 1996. *Man and Microbes: Disease and Plagues in History and Modern Times.* New York: Simon and Schuster/Touchstone.

Kidder, Tracy. 2004. *Mountains Beyond Mountains: The Story of Dr. Paul Farmer, the Man Who Would Cure the World.* New York: Random House.

Mack, Arien, ed. 1991. *In Time of Plague: The History and Social Consequences of Lethal Epidemic Disease.* New York: New York University Press.

Markel, Howard. 2004. *When Germs Travel.* New York: Vintage.

Office of Public Health and Science (OPHS): http://www.hhs.gov/ophs/index.html.

Office of the Surgeon General (OSG): http://www.surgeongeneral.gov/.

SOCIAL/CULTURAL ASPECTS

Bull, Chris, ed. *While the World Sleeps: Writing from the First Twenty Years of the Global AIDS Plague.* New York: Thunder's Mouth Press.

Fee, Elizabeth, and Daniel M. Fox, eds. 1988. *AIDS: The Burdens of History.* Berkeley: University of California Press.

Lemelle, Anthony J., Jr, Allen J. Leblanc, and Charlene Harrington. 1999. *Readings in the Sociology of AIDS.* Upper Saddle River, NJ: Prentice-Hall.

Huber, Joan, and Beth Schneider, eds. 1991. *The Social Context of AIDS.* Thousand Oaks, CA: Sage.

Kane, Stephanie. 1998. *AIDS Alibis: Sex, Drugs, and Crime in the Americas.* Philadelphia: Temple University Press.

Pollak, Micheal, with Genevieve Paicheler and Janine Pierret. 1992. *AIDS: A Problem for Sociological Research.* London: Sage.

Roleff, T.L., ed. *AIDS: Opposing Viewpoints.* Farmington Hills, MI: Greenhaven Press.

Sontag, Susan. 1989. *AIDS and Its Metaphors.* New York: Farrar, Straus and Giroux.

Treichler, Paula A. 1999. *How to Have Theory in an Epidemic: Cultural Chronicles of AIDS*. Durham: Duke University Press.
Wyatt-Morley, Catherine. 1997. *AIDS Memoir: Journal of an HIV Positive Mother*. Kumarian Press.

Specific Populations
Children

Guest, Emma. 2001. *Children of AIDS: Africa's Orphan Crisis*. Scottsville, South Africa: Pluto Press.
Kirp, David L. 1989. *Learning by Heart: AIDS and School Children in America's Communities*. New Brunswick, NJ: Rutgers University Press.

Drug Users

Friedman, Samuel R. Richard Curtis, Alan Neaigus, Benny Jose, and Don C. Des Jarlais. 1999. *Social Networks, Drug Injectors' Lives, and HIV/AIDS*. New York: Springer.
Malinowska-Sempruch, Kasia, and Sarah Gallagher. 2004. *War on Drugs, HIV/AIDS, and Human Rights*. New York: International Debate Education Association.

GLBT

Aggleton, P., ed. 1996. *Bisexualities and AIDS: International Perspectives*. Bristol, PA: Taylor and Francis.
Bockting, W. and Sheila Kirk, eds. 2001. *Transgender and HIV: Risks, Prevention, and Care*. New York: Haworth.
Dowsett, Gary W. 1996. *Practicing Desire: Homosexual Sex in the Era of AIDS*. Stanford, CA: Stanford University Press.
Levine, Martin et al., eds. 1997. *In Changing Times: Gay Men and Lesbians Encounter HIV/AIDS*. University of Chicago Press.
Stoller, Nancy. 1998. *Lessons from the Damned: Queers, Whores, and Junkies Respond to AIDS*. New York: Routledge.

Men

Foreman, Martin. 1999. *AIDS and Men: Taking Risks or Taking Responsibility?* London: Zed Books.
Simpson, Anthony. 2009. *Boys to Men in the Shadow of AIDS: Masculinities and HIV Risk in Zambia*. New York: Palgrave Macmillan.

Prisoners

Lines, R. 2002. "Pros and Cons: A Guide to Creating Successful Community Based HIV/AIDS Programs for Prisoners. Toronto: Pagan, Prisoners HIV/AIDS Support Action Network." International Conference on AIDS. July 7–12; 14: abstract no. G12738.

The Members of the ACE Program of the Bedford Hills Correctional Facility. 1998. *Breaking the Walls of Silence: AIDS and Women in a New York State Maximum-Security Prison*. Overlook Press.

Racial/Ethnic Minorities

Cohen, Cathy. *The Boundaries of Blackness: AIDS and the Breakdown of Black Politics*. Chicago: University of Chicago. 1999.

White, Renee T. 1999. *Putting Risk in Perspective: Black Teenage Lives in the Era of AIDS*. Lanham: Rowman and Littlefield Publishers, Inc.

Women

Boehmer, Ulrike. 2000. *The Personal and the Political: Women's Activism in Response to the Breast Cancer and AIDS Epidemic*. Albany, NY: State University of New York.

Campbell, C.A. 1999. *Women, Families, and HIV/AIDS: A Sociological Perspective on the Epidemic in America*. New York: Cambridge.

Ciambrone, Desiree. 2003. *Women's Experiences with HIV/AIDS: Mending Fractured Selves*. New York: Haworth.

Corea, Gena. 1992. *The Invisible Epidemic: The Story of Women and AIDS*. New York: HarperCollins.

Farmer, Paul, Margaret Conners, and Janie Simmons, eds. 1996. *Women, Poverty, and AIDS: Sex, Drugs and Structural Violence*. Monroe, ME: Common Courage Press.

Goldstein and Manlow, eds. 1997. *The Gender Politics of HIV/AIDS in Women*. New York University Press.

Hogan, Kagie. 2001. *Women Take Care: Gender, Race, and the Culture of AIDS*. Ithaca, NY: Cornell University Press.

Kurth, Ann. 1993. *Until the Cure: Caring for Women with HIV*. New Haven, CT: Yale University Press.

Lather, Patti, and Chris Smithies. 1997. *Troubling the Angels: Women Living with HIV/AIDS*. Boulder, CO: Westview Press.

Schneider, Beth. 1995. *Women Resisting AIDS*. Philadelphia: Temple University Press.

Sobo, Elisa J. 1995. *Choosing Unsafe Sex: AIDS Risk Denial among Disadvantaged Women*. Philadelphia: University of Pennsylvania Press.

VACCINES

Cohen, Jon. 2001. *A Shot in the Dark: The Wayward Search for an AIDS Vaccine*. W.W. Norton.

International AIDS Vaccine Initiative (IAVI): http://www.iavi.org/.

Kahn, Patricia, ed. 2005. *AIDS Vaccine Handbook: Global Perspectives*. New York: AIDS Vaccine Advisory Coalition.

INDEX

Note: Page numbers followed by a p indicate the references are to a picture.

Nucleoside/nucleotide RT inhibitors
(NRTIs, "nukes"), 41–42
Nureyev, Rudolf, 179

Obama, U.S. President Barack, 54p,
55, 88, 188
Office of AIDS Research (OAR),
177, 216
Office of HIV/AIDS Policy (OHAP),
216
Office of Public Health and Science
(OPHS), 216
Office of the Surgeon General (OSG),
216
Older adults. *See* Elderly
Opportunistic infections, 6, 38, 67,
180
Oral HIV testing, 55–57, 179, 182,
185
Orphan Drug Act, 173
Outkast, 101

Pacific islanders, 51, 185
Pandemic, 3
defined, 7
Peace Corps, 85
Pediatric AIDS Foundation, 177
Pediatric HIV/AIDS, 110
PEPFAR (U.S. President's
Emergency Plan for AIDS
Relief), 54–55, 87–88, 184,
185, 187
Perinatal transmission, 116, 138, 172,
194, 208–209. *See also*
Pregnancy
preventing 39–40, 45, 46, 50, 51,
53, 179, 206
Perth Group, 37
Peru, 53
Phambili clinical trials, 45
Pharmaceutical development, 69. *See
also* Drug development
process
Philadelphia (film), 105, 179

Phir Milenge ("We Will Meet Again,"
Indian film), 105
Piercing, body, 144
Pneumocystis carinii pneumonia, 6,
8, 191–193
Pneumonia, 6, 8
Policy, 75–79, 81–88, 216, 217. *See
also* Appendix A Timeline;
Politics and political issues;
Reagan, U.S. President
Ronald; *specific political fig-
ures, specific legislation*
Politics and political issues, 50,
55–56, 57, 65–66, 69, 91,
102–105, 136, 145. *See also*
Appendix A Timeline; Pol-
icy; Reagan, U.S. President
Ronald; *specific political fig-
ures, specific legislation*
Polymerase Chain Reaction (PCR)
testing, 56
Pope Benedict XVI, 188
Popular culture, 97–107
Portugal, 184
Postnatal, 112
Poverty, 45, 52–53, 69, 117, 125,
137–138, 160, 183, 187
Powell, Colin, 183
Pregnancy, 10, 39–40, 51, 109–111,
194, 212
Prenatal, 112
Presidential Advisory Council on
HIV/AIDS, 180
Prevention, 10, 12, 15–18, 28, 31, 33,
49–57, 66, 75–76, 78, 82,
92, 111–112, 144, 145,
152–155, 157, 161, 183,
184, 187, 194–198
and media, 53–55
among youth, 119
Prezista, 44
Prisons, 159–161, 165–167, 179, 180,
206
(PRODUCT) RED, 101, 186

ABOUT THE AUTHORS

Kathy S. Stolley, PhD, is Batten Associate Professor of Sociology and Coordinator of Women's and Gender Studies at Virginia Wesleyan College in Norfolk, Virginia. Her emphasis is applied sociology—using sociological tools and perspectives to bring about positive social change. She is recipient of her college's 2009 distinguished teaching award. In addition to teaching, she has worked in various sociological practice positions outside of academics, including policing, organizational consulting, and social science research. Dr. Stolley was editor-in-chief of the applied sociology journal, *Social Insight: Knowledge at Work*, and her research has been published in various professional journals. She is also the author of *The Basics of Sociology* (2005) and coeditor of the two-volume *Praeger Handbook of Adoption* (2006).

John E. Glass is Professor of Sociology at Collin County Community College, Frisco, Texas. He holds a PhD in Sociology from the University of North Texas. His current areas of interest include developing a behaviorological approach to sociology, creating more effective pedagogical techniques to the teaching of sociology, and volunteering with international NGOs working in developing countries to improve educational opportunities for their citizens. Prior to teaching full-time, he worked in the field of substance abuse as a counselor, trainer, Programs Director and Facility Director and in the field of domestic violence as Director of Program Evaluation. He has served on the boards of the Sociological Practice Association and the Society for Applied Sociology and is now serving on the executive team of Behaviorists for Social Responsibility.